Preparatory
EMS Systems

AEMT Education Standard

Applies fundamental knowledge of the EMS system, safety/well-being of the AEMT, medical/legal and ethical issues to the provision of emergency care.

AEMT-Level Instructional Guideline

The AEMT Instructional Guidelines in this section include all the topics and material at the EMT level PLUS the following material:

I. Quality Improvement
    A. System for Continually Evaluating and Improving Care
    B. Continuous Quality Improvement (CQI)
    C. Dynamic Process

II. Patient Safety
    A. Significant – One of The Most Urgent Health Care Challenges
    B. Incidence-IOM Report "To Err Is Human" Up to 98,000 Patients Die Due to Medical Errors
    C. High-Risk Activities
        1. Hand off
        2. Communication issues
        3. Medication issues
        4. Airway issues
        5. Dropping patients
        6. Ambulance crashes
        7. Spinal immobilization
    D. How Errors Happen
        1. Skills based failure
        2. Rules based failure
        3. Knowledge based failure
    E. Preventing Errors
        1. Environmental
            a. Clear protocols
            b. Light
            c. Minimal interruptions
            d. Organization and packaging of drugs
        2. Individual
            a. Reflection in action
            b. Constantly question assumptions
            c. Reflection bias

            d.   Use decision aids
            e.   Ask for help

III.   Education
        A.   Levels of EMS licensure
        B.   National EMS Education Agenda for the Future: A Systems Approach

IV.   Authorization to Practice
        A.   Legislative Decisions on Scope of Practice
        B.   State EMS Office Oversight
        C.   Medical Oversight
                1.   Clinical
                        a.   Offline Protocols
                        b.   Online Protocols
                        c.   Standing orders
                2.   Quality improvement
                3.   Administrative
        D.   Local Credentialing
        E.   Employer Policies and Procedures

V.   Integration With Other Professionals and Continuity of Care
        A.   Medical Personnel
        B.   Law Enforcement
        C.   Emergency Management
        D.   Home Healthcare Providers
        E.   Other Responders

VI.   Maintenance of Certification and Licensure
        A.   Personal Responsibility
        B.   Continuing Education
        C.   Skill Competency Verification
        D.   Criminal Implications
        E.   Fees

Preparatory
Research

AEMT Education Standard

Applies fundamental knowledge of the EMS system, safety/well-being of the AEMT, medical/legal and ethical issues to the provision of emergency care.

AEMT-Level Instructional Guideline

The AEMT Instructional Guidelines in this section include all the topics and material at the EMT level.

Preparatory
Workforce Safety and Wellness

AEMT Education Standard

Applies fundamental knowledge of the EMS system, safety/well-being of the AEMT, medical/legal and ethical issues to the provision of emergency care.

AEMT-Level Instructional Guideline

The AEMT Instructional Guidelines in this section include all the topics and material at the EMT level.

Preparatory
Documentation

AEMT Education Standard

Applies fundamental knowledge of the EMS system, safety/well-being of the AEMT, medical/legal and ethical issues to the provision of emergency care.

AEMT-Level Instructional Guideline

The AEMT Instructional Guidelines in this section include all the topics and material at the EMT level PLUS the following material:

I.   Principles of Medical Documentation and Report Writing
   A.   Minimum Data Set
      1.   Patient information
         a.   Chief complaint
         b.   Initial assessment
         c.   Vital signs
         d.   Patient Demographics
      2.   Administrative information
         a.   Time incident reported
         b.   Time unit notified
         c.   Time of arrival at patient
         d.   Time unit left scene
         e.   Time of arrival at destination
         f.   Time of transfer of care
      3.   Accurate and synchronous clocks
   B.   Prehospital Care Report
      1.   Functions
         a.   Continuity of care
         b.   Legal document
         c.   Educational
         d.   Administrative
            i.   billing
            ii.   service statistics
         e.   Research
         f.   Evaluation and continuous quality improvement
      2.   Uses
         a.   Types
            i.   traditional written form with check boxes and a section for narrative
            ii.   computerized version where information is filled in by means of an electronic device or over the Internet

b. Sections
   i. run data
   ii. patient data
   iii. check boxes
   iv. narrative section
      a) systems documentation
      b) SOAPE format
c. Confidentiality
d. Distribution
e. Health Information Portability and Accountability Act of 1996 (HIPAA)

3. Falsification Issues

C. Documentation of Patient Refusal
1. Before leaving the scene
   a. Document patient's able to make a rational, informed decision
   b. Inform the patient why he should go and what may happen to him if he does not
   c. Consult medical direction as directed by local protocol
   d. Document any assessment
   e. Obtain appropriate witness signature
   f. Complete the prehospital care report
      i. care patient refused
      ii. statement that the EMT explained to the patient the possible consequences of failure to accept care, including potential death
      iii. offer alternative methods of gaining care
      iv. state willingness to return

D. Special Situations/Reports/Incident Reporting
1. Correction of errors
   a. Errors discovered while the report form is being hand written
   b. Errors discovered after a hand written report form is submitted
   c. Errors discovered while/after completing an electronic report
2. Multiple Casualty Incidents (MCI)
   a. When there is not enough time to complete the form before the next call, the EMT will need to fill out the report later
   b. The local MCI plan should have some means of recording important medical information temporarily
   c. The standard for completing the form in an MCI is not the same as for a typical call
3. Special situation reports
   a. Used to document events that should be reported to local authorities, or to amplify and supplement primary report
   b. Should be submitted in timely manner and should include the names of all agencies, people, and facilities involved
   c. The report, and copies if appropriate, should be submitted to the authority described by local protocol

d. Exposure
e. Injury
f. Goal should be to provide a report prior to departing from the hospital
g. The EMT should keep a copy of this transfer report for use as a reference during the primary prehospital care report and should submit the copy with the final prehospital care report

Preparatory
EMS System Communication

AEMT Education Standard

Applies fundamental knowledge of the EMS system, safety/well-being of the AEMT, medical/legal and ethical issues to the provision of emergency care.

AEMT-Level Instructional Guideline

The AEMT Instructional Guidelines in this section include all the topics and material at the EMT level PLUS the following material:

I.   EMS Communication System
    A.   System Components
        1.   Base station
        2.   Mobile radios (transmitter/receivers)
            a.   Vehicular mounted device
            b.   Mobile transmitters usually transmit at lower power than base stations (typically 20 to 50 watts)
            c.   Typical transmission range is 10 to 15 miles over average terrain
        3.   Portable radios (transmitter/receivers)
            a.   Handheld device
            b.   Typically have power output of 1 to 5 watts, limiting their range
        4.   Repeater/base station
        5.   Digital radio equipment
        6.   Cellular telephones
    B.   Radio Communications
        1.   Radio frequencies
        2.   Response to the scene
            a.   The dispatcher needs to be notified that the call was received
            b.   Dispatch needs to know that the unit is en route
        3.   Arrival at the scene
        4.   Depart the scene
            a.   Dispatcher must be notified
            b.   Prolonged on scene times with absence of communications
        5.   Arrival at the receiving facility or rendezvous point
        6.   Arrival for service after patient transfer

II.   Communicating With Other Health Care Professionals
    A.   Communication With Medical Control
        1.   Medical control is at the receiving facility. Medical control is at a separate site

2. AEMTs may need to contact medical control for consultation and to get orders for administration of medications
3. AEMTs must be accurate
4. After receiving an order for a medication or procedure—repeat the order back word for word
5. Orders that are unclear or appear to be inappropriate should be questioned or clarified for the AEMT

B. Communication With Receiving Facilities
1. AEMT having the right room, equipment and personnel prepared or allow the facility to plan for the patient
2. Patient reporting concepts
    a. When speaking on the radio, keep these principles in mind:
        i. make sure the radio is on and volume is properly adjusted
        ii. listen to the frequency and ensure it is clear before beginning a transmission
        iii. press the "press to talk" (ptt) button on the radio and wait for one second before speaking
        iv. speak with lips about 2 to 3 inches from the microphone
        v. address the unit being called, and then give the name of the unit
        vi. the unit being called will signal that the transmission should start
        vii. speak clearly, calmly, and slowly in a monotone voice
        viii. keep transmissions brief
        ix. use clear text
        x. avoid codes or agency specific terms
        xi. avoid meaningless phrases like "be advised"
        xii. courtesy is assumed, one should limit saying "please," "thank you," and "you're welcome"
        xiii. when transmitting a number that might be confused (e.g. a number in the teens), give the number, then give the individual digits
        xiv. the airwaves are public and scanners are popular
        xv. remain objective and impartial in describing patients
        xvi. do not use profanity on the air
        xvii. avoid words that are difficult to hear like "yes" and "no"; use "affirmative" and "negative"
        xviii. use the standard format for transmission of information
        xix. when the transmission is finished, indicate this by saying "over"
        xx. avoid offering a diagnosis of the patient's problem
        xxi. use EMS frequencies only for EMS communication
        xxii. reduce background noise
    b. Notify the dispatcher when the unit leaves the scene

   c. When communicating with medical direction or the receiving facility, a verbal report should be given. The essential elements of such a report, in an order that is efficient and effective, are:

     i. identify unit and level of provider (can utilize the name of the provider giving the report as well as the unit identification)

     ii. estimated time of arrival

     iii. current patient condition

     iv. patient's age and sex

     v. mental status

     vi. chief complaint

     vii. brief, pertinent history of the present illness

     viii. major past illnesses

     ix. baseline vital signs

     x. pertinent findings of the physical exam

     xi. emergency medical care given

     xii. response to emergency medical care

   d. After giving this information, the AEMT will continue to assess the patient

   e. Arrival at the hospital

     i. the dispatcher must be notified

     ii. in some systems, the hospital should also be notified

   f. Leaving the hospital for the station

   g. Arrival at the station

 C. System Maintenance

  1. Communication equipment needs to be checked to ensure that a radio is not drifting form its assigned frequency

  2. As technology changes, new equipment becomes available that may have a role in EMS systems

  3. AEMT need to be able to consult on-line medical direction, and EMS system must provide back-up

 D. Phone/Cellular Communications

  1. Should be treated similar to radio communications when it comes to content and strategies for delivery of pertinent information

  2. The AEMT should be familiar with important and commonly utilized telephone numbers, such as medical control, local hospital Emergency Departments, dispatch centers

  3. The AEMT should also have a familiarity with cellular technologies and knowledge of the location of cellular dead spots in the area

  4. There should be another plan for when a cellular transmission fail during a report or communication with another agency

III. Team Communication and Dynamics

Preparatory
Therapeutic Communication

AEMT Education Standard

Applies fundamental knowledge of the EMS system, safety/well-being of the AEMT, medical/legal and ethical issues to the provision of emergency care.

AEMT-Level Instructional Guideline

The AEMT Instructional Guidelines in this section include all the topics and material at the EMT level PLUS the following material:

I.   Principles of Communicating With Patients in a Manner That Achieves a Positive Relationship
    A.   Dealing With Difficult Patients
    B.   Most Patients Are More Than Willing to Talk
        1.   Difficult interviews
        2.   Techniques to use
            a.   Start the interview in the normal manner.
            b.   Attempt to use open-ended questions
            c.   Provide positive feedback
            d.   Make sure the patient understands the questions
            e.   Continue to ask questions
        3.   Interviewing a hostile patient
        4.   Hearing impaired patients
        5.   Patients under the influence of street drugs or alcohol
        6.   Sexually aggressive patients

Preparatory
Medical/Legal and Ethics

AEMT Education Standard

Applies fundamental knowledge of the EMS system, safety/well-being of the AEMT, medical/legal and ethical issues to the provision of emergency care.

AEMT-Level Instructional Guideline

The AEMT Instructional Guidelines in this section include all the topics and material at the EMT level.

Anatomy and Physiology

Anatomy and Physiology

AEMT Education Standard

Integrates complex knowledge of the anatomy and physiology of the airway, respiratory and circulatory systems to the practice of EMS.

AEMT-Level Instructional Guideline

The AEMT Instructional Guidelines in this section include all the topics and material at the EMT level, PLUS the following material:

I. Anatomy and Body Functions
   A. Anatomical Planes
      1. Frontal or coronal plane
      2. Sagittal or lateral plane
      3. Transverse or axial plane
   B. Standard Anatomic Terms
   C. Body Systems
      1. Skeletal
         a. Components
            i.   skull
            ii.   face
            iii. vertebral column
            iv.   thorax
            v.   pelvis
            vi.   upper extremities
            vii. lower extremities
         b. Joints
         c. Function
      2. Muscular
         a. Types
            i.   skeletal
            ii.   smooth
            iii. cardiac
         b. Function
   D. Respiratory System
      1. General function of the respiratory system
         a. Upper respiratory tract
         b. Lower respiratory tract
      2. Structure and functions of the nasal cavities and pharynx
         a. Nasal cavities
            i.   nose

          ii.   nasal cavities
          iii.   nasal septum
          iv.   nasal mucosa
          v.   olfactory receptors
          vi.   paranasal sinuses

- b. Pharynx
    - i. nasopharynx
    - ii. soft palate
    - iii. oropharynx
    - iv. laryngopharynx

3. Structure and function of the larynx and the speaking mechanism
   a. Voice box
   b. Thyroid cartilage
   c. Epiglottis
   d. Vocal cords
   e. Glottis

4. Structure and functions of the trachea and bronchial tree
   a. Trachea
   b. Primary bronchi
   c. Bronchial tree
   d. Right and left main-stem bronchi
   e. Bronchioles

5. Lungs
   a. Location and function
   b. Pleural membranes
      i. parietal pleura
      ii. visceral pleura
      iii. serous fluid
   c. Hilus

6. Structure and function of the alveoli and pulmonary capillaries

7. Mechanism of breathing
   a. Mechanical ventilation
      i. mechanism of inhalation
         a) inspiration
         b) phrenic nerve
         c) intercostal nerves
         d) respiration
         e) ventilation/perfusion disturbance
         f) diaphragm
         g) external intercostal muscles
         h) internal intercostal muscles
         i) pressures
      ii. changes in air pressure that occur within the thoracic cavity during respiration
         a) atmospheric
         b) intrapleural
         c) intrapulmonic

        b.   Role of the visceral and parietal pleura in respiration
        c.   Mechanics of exhalation
  8.   Explain the diffusion of gases in external and internal respiration
  9.   Discuss pulmonary volumes
        a.   Tidal volume
        b.   Minute respiratory volume (MRV)
        c.   Vital capacity
  10.   Physiological dead space and lung compliance
  11.   Oxygen and carbon dioxide transport in the blood
  12.   Nervous and chemical mechanisms that regulate respiration
  13.   Respiration and acid-base balance
        a.   Respiratory acidosis and alkalosis
        b.   Metabolic acidosis and alkalosis

E.   Circulatory
  1.   Blood
        a.   Composition and function of blood
        b.   Composition and function of blood plasma
              i.   amount
              ii.   color
              iii.   pH
              iv.   viscosity
              v.   plasma
        c.   Primary hemopoietic tissue
        d.   Function of red blood cells
        e.   Red blood cell production in hypoxic state
        f.   Red blood cell and hemoglobin destruction
        g.   ABO group and Rh factor blood types
        h.   Function of white blood cells (leukocytes)
        i.   Platelets
  2.   The heart
        a.   Location and features of the heart
              i.   mediastinum
              ii.   pericardial membranes
              iii.   fibrous pericardium
              iv.   parietal pericardium
              v.   epicardium
        b.   Chambers of the heart
              i.   myocardium
              ii.   endocardium
              iii.   right and left atria
              iv.   right and left ventricles
        c.   Valves of the heart and their function
              i.   tricuspid valve
              ii.   bicuspid valve (mitral valve)
              iii.   aortic valve
              iv.   pulmonary semilunar valve

    d. Cardiac cycle

    e. Coronary Arteries

    f. Major blood vessels

    g. Stroke volume, cardiac output, and Starling's law of he heart

    h. Nervous system regulation of the function of the heart

  3. Blood vessels and circulation

    a. Structure and function of the blood vessels, arteries, veins and capillaries

    b. Arterial and venous anastomosis

    c. Structure of capillaries

    d. Exchange of gases that occurs at the capillary level

    e. Mechanism that regulate blood flow through arteries, capillaries, and veins

    f. Pathway and purpose of the pulmonary circulation

    g. Pathway of the systemic circulation

    h. Pathway and purpose of the hepatic portal circulation

    i. Branches of the aorta and their distributions

    j. Major systemic arteries and the parts of the body they nourish

    k. Major systemic veins and the parts of the body they drain of blood

    l. Hemodynamics

      i. blood pressure

        a) venous return

        b) pulse pressure

        c) peripheral resistance

      ii. factors that maintain systemic blood pressure

        a) heart rate and force of contraction

        b) vessel elasticity

        c) blood viscosity

        d) hormones

        e) peripheral resistance

      iii. osmosis

      iv. diffusion

      v. facilitated diffusion

      vi. active transport

      vii. hydrostatic pressure

      viii. oncotic pressure

    m. Regulation of blood pressure by the heart and kidneys

    n. Medulla and autonomic nervous system regulation of the diameter of the blood vessels

    o. Coordination of the cardiac, vasomotor, and respiratory centers to control blood flow through the tissues

F. Nervous System

  1. Structural division

    a. Central nervous system (CNS)

      i. brain

      ii. spinal cord

    b. Peripheral nervous system (PNS)

2. Functional
   a. Autonomic
      i. sympathetic
      ii. parasympathetic
3. Functions of the nervous system
   a. Consciousness
      i. cerebral hemispheres
      ii. reticular activating system (center of consciousness)
   b. Sensory function
   c. Motor function
   d. Fight-or-flight response

G. Integumentary (Skin)
   1. Structures
      a. Epidermis
      b. Dermis
      c. Subcutaneous layer
   2. Functions of the skin
      a. Protection
      b. Temperature control

H. Digestive System
   1. Structures
      a. Esophagus
      b. Stomach
      c. Intestines
      d. Liver
      e. Pancreas

I. Endocrine System
   1. Structures
      a. Pancreas
      b. Adrenal glands
         i. epinephrine
         ii. norepinephrine
   2. Function
      a. Control of blood glucose level
      b. Stimulate sympathetic nervous system

J. Renal System
   1. Structures
      a. Kidneys
      b. Bladder
      c. Urethra
   2. Function
      a. Blood filtration
      b. Fluid balance
      c. Buffer

K. Reproductive System
   1. Male
      a. Structures

     i. testicles

     ii. penis

   b. Functions

     i. reproduction

     ii. urination

     iii. hormones

  2. Female

   a. Structures

     i. ovaries

     ii. fallopian tubes

     iii. uterus

     iv. vagina

   b. Functions

     i. reproduction

     ii. hormones

II. Life Support Chain

  A. Fundamental Elements

   1. Oxygenation

    a. Alveolar/capillary gas exchange

    b. Cell/capillary gas exchange

   2. Perfusion

    a. Oxygen

    b. Glucose

    c. Removal of carbon dioxide and other waste products

   3. Cell environment

    a. Aerobic metabolism

     i. high atp (energy) production

     ii. byproduct of water and carbon dioxide

    b. Anaerobic metabolism

     i. low atp (energy) production

     ii. byproduct of lactic acid

  B. Issues Affecting Fundamental Elements

   1. Composition of ambient air

   2. Patency of the airway

   3. Mechanics of ventilation

   4. Regulation of respiration

   5. Ventilation/perfusion ratio

   6. Transport of gases

   7. Blood volume

   8. Effectiveness of the heart as a pump

   9. Vessel size and resistance (systemic vascular resistance)

   10. Effects of acid on cells and organs

III. Age-Related Variations for Pediatrics and Geriatrics

  A. See Special Patient Populations

Medical Terminology

AEMT Education Standard

Uses foundational anatomical and medical terms and abbreviations in written and oral communication with colleagues and other health care professional.

AEMT-Level Instructional Guideline

The AEMT Instructional Guidelines in this section include all the topics and material at the EMT level.

Pathophysiology
Pathophysiology

AEMT Education Standard

Applies comprehensive knowledge of the pathophysiology of respiration and perfusion to patient assessment and management.

AEMT-Level Instructional Guideline

The AEMT Instructional Guidelines in this section include all the topics and material at the EMT level, PLUS the following material:

I.   Introduction
    A.   Correlation Of Pathophysiology With Disease Process
        1.   Cells and the multi-cellular organism
        2.   Cellular communication

II.   Basic Cellular Review
    A.   Major Classes of Cells
    B.   Chief Cellular Functions
    C.   Cellular Components
        1.   Structure
        2.   Function

III.   Alteration in Cells and Tissues

IV.   Cellular Injury
    A.   Hypoxic Injury - Causes
        1.   Decreased oxygenation
        2.   Loss of hemoglobin or hemoglobin function
        3.   Decreased red blood cells
        4.   Respiratory or cardiovascular system disease

V.   Hypoperfusion
    A.   Pathogenesis
        1.   Decreased cardiac output
        2.   Compensatory mechanisms
            a.   Catecholamine release
                i.   epinephrine
                ii.   norepinephrine
                iii.   increase in systemic vascular resistance
                    a)   increased blood volume
                    b)   vasoconstriction

              iv.   increased stroke volume
              v.   increased heart rate
              vi.   increased preload

3.   Oxygen impairment
     a.   Anaerobic metabolism
     b.   Increased lactate
     c.   Metabolic acidosis
          i.   decreased oxygen affinity for hemoglobin
          ii.   decreased atp
          iii.   changes in cellular electrolytes
          iv.   cellular edema
          v.   release of lysosomal enzymes
     d.   Impaired glucose use

B.   Types of Shock
1.   Cardiogenic shock
     a.   Defined
     b.   Pathophysiology
     c.   Evaluation and treatment
2.   Hypovolemic shock
     a.   Defined
     b.   Pathophysiology
     c.   Evaluation and treatment
3.   Neurogenic shock
     a.   Defined
     b.   Pathophysiology
     c.   Evaluation and treatment
4.   Anaphylactic shock
     a.   Defined
     b.   Pathophysiology
     c.   Evaluation and treatment
5.   Septic shock
     a.   Defined
     b.   Pathophysiology
     c.   Evaluation and treatment

Life Span Development
Life Span Development

AEMT Education Standard

Applies fundamental knowledge of life span development to patient assessment and management.

AEMT-Level Instructional Guideline

The AEMT Instructional Guidelines in this section include all the topics and material at the EMT level.

Public Health
Public Health

Public Health

AEMT Education Standard

Uses simple knowledge of the principles of the role of EMS during public health emergencies.

AEMT-Level Instructional Guideline

The AEMT Instructional Guidelines in this section include all the topics and material at the EMT level, PLUS the following material:

I. Basic Principles of Public Health
    A. Role of Public Health
        1. Many definitions
        2. Public health mission and functions
        3. Public health differs from individual patient care
        4. Review accomplishments of public health
            a. Widespread vaccinations
            b. Clean drinking water and sewage systems
            c. Declining infectious disease
            d. Fluoridated water
            e. Reduction in use of tobacco products
            f. Prenatal care
            g. Others
    B. Public Health Laws, Regulations and Guidelines
    C. EMS Interface With Public Health
        1. EMS is a public health system
            a. EMS provides a critical public health function
            b. Incorporate public health services into EMS system
            c. Collaborations with other public health agencies
        2. Roles for EMS in public health
            a. Health prevention and promotion
                i. primary prevention—preventing disease development
                    a) vaccination
                    b) education
                ii. secondary prevention—preventing the complications and/or progression of disease
                iii. health screenings
            b. Disease surveillance
                i. EMS providers are first line care givers
                ii. patient care reports may provide information on epidemics of disease

3.   Injury prevention
     a.   Safety equipment
     b.   Education
          i.   car seat safety
          ii.   seat belt use
          iii.   helmet use
          iv.   driving under the influence
          v.   falls
          vi.   fire
     c.   Injury surveillance
D.   Role of EMS in Public Health Emergencies
     1.   Types of public health emergencies
     2.   EMS response

Pharmacology
Principles of Pharmacology

Applies (to patient assessment and management) fundamental knowledge of the medications carried by AEMTs that may be administered to a patient during an emergency.

AEMT-Level Instructional Guideline

The AEMT Instructional Guidelines in this section include all the topics and material at the EMT level PLUS the following material:

I.   Medication Safety

II.   Medication Legislation
      A.   Pure Food and Drug Act
      B.   Federal Food, Drug and Cosmetic Act
      C.   Harrison Narcotic Act
      D.   Controlled Substances Act
      E.   Drug Enforcement Agency
      F.   Development of Pharmaceuticals
            1.   Food and Drug Administration approval process
            2.   Special Considerations
                  a.   Pregnancy
                  b.   Pediatrics
                  c.   Geriatrics
      G.   Drug Forms
            1.   Liquids
            2.   Solids
            3.   Gases

III.   Naming
      A.   Chemical
      B.   Generic
      C.   Propriety/Trade
      D.   Official
      E.   Authoritative Sources of Drug Information
            1.   United States Pharmacopeia (USP)
            2.   Physician's Desk Reference (PDR)
            3.   Drug package inserts
            4.   Drug handbooks

IV.   Classifications
    A.   Body System Affected
    B.   Class of Agent
    C.   Classifications by Body System
        1.   Central nervous system
            a.   Autonomic pharmacology
                i.   cholinergics
                ii.   anticholinergic drug definitions
                iii.   adrenergics
                iv.   antiadrenergic
                    a)   alpha – adrenergic blockers
                    b)   beta – adrenergic blockers
            b.   Analgesics
                i.   opioid agonists
                ii.   opioid antagonists
                iii.   non steroidal anti – inflammatory drugs
            c.   Sedative/hypnotic
                i.   benzodiazepines
                ii.   barbiturates
            d.   Anticonvulsants
            e.   Stimulants
        2.   Cardiovascular drug definitions
            a.   Anti-dysrhythmics
            b.   Cardiac glycosides
            c.   Antihypertensives
            d.   Antianginal drugs
        3.   Drugs affecting the blood
        4.   Psychiatric medications
        5.   Respiratory system
            a.   Mucolytics
            b.   Cholinergic antagonists
            c.   Sympathomimetics
            d.   Xanthine derivatives
            e.   Antihistamines
        6.   Endocrine system -- drugs affecting the pancreas
            a.   Insulin preparations
            b.   Oral hypoglycemic agents
            c.   Hyperglycemic agents
        7.   Herbal preparations
            a.   Potential Implications
                i.   interaction with pharmaceuticals
                ii.   idiosyncratic reactions
                iii.   manufacturing error
                iv.   contamination
                v.   substitution

          b.   Adulteration
               i.   incorrect preparation
               ii.   incorrect labeling
   8.   Over the counter medications
          a.   Drugs affecting the central nervous system
               i.   sedatives
               ii.   stimulants
               iii.   hallucinogenic (dextromethorophan)
          b.   Drugs affecting the respiratory system
               i.   asthma treatment products
               ii.   cold and allergy products
          c.   Supplements
               i.   herbs
               ii.   vitamins
               iii.   minerals
               iv.   other

V.   Storage and Security
    A.   Factors Affecting Drug Potency
         1.   Temperature
         2.   Light
         3.   Moisture
         4.   Shelf Life
    B.   Locking and Double Locking of Medications

VI.   Drug Terminology
    A.   Antagonism
    B.   Bolus
    C.   Contraindications
    D.   Cumulative Action
    E.   Depressant
    F.   Habituation
    G.   Hypersensitivity
    H.   Idiosyncrasy
    I.   Indication
    J.   Potentiation
    K.   Refractory
    L.   Side Effects
    M.   Stimulant
    N.   Synergism
    O.   Therapeutic Action
    P.   Tolerance
    Q.   Untoward Effect

VII.   Pharmacological Concepts
    A.   Pharmacokinetics
        1.   Absorption
        2.   Distribution
        3.   Biotransformation
        4.   Metabolism and Excretion -- organs of elimination
            a.   kidneys
            b.   intestine
            c.   lungs
            d.   exocrine glands
    B.   Pharmacodynamics
        1.   Mechanism of action
            a.   Drug receptor interaction
                i.   agonists
                ii.   antagonists
                iii.   affinity
                iv.   efficacy
            b.   Drug enzyme interaction
        2.   Medication response relationship
            a.   Plasma levels
            b.   Biologic half–life
            c.   Therapeutic threshold
            d.   Therapeutic index
            e.   LD 50
            f.   Factors altering drug response
                i.   age
                ii.   sex
                iii.   body mass index
                iv.   pathologic state
                v.   genetic factors
                vi.   time of administration
                vii.   psychological factors
                viii.   predictable responses
                    a)   tolerance
                    b)   cross tolerance
                ix.   iatrogenic responses\
                x.   drug allergy
                xi.   anaphylactic reaction
                xii.   delayed reaction ("serum sickness")
                xiii.   hypersensitivity
                xiv.   idiosyncrasy
                xv.   cumulative effect
                xvi.   drug dependence
                xvii.   drug antagonism
                xviii.   summation (addition or additive effect)
                xix.   synergism

          xx.   potentiation
          xxi.   interference
3.   Medication interaction
4.   Toxicity

Pharmacology
Medication Administration

Applies (to patient assessment and management) fundamental knowledge of the medications carried by AEMTs that may be administered to a patient during an emergency.

AEMT-Level Instructional Guideline

The AEMT Instructional Guidelines in this section include all the topics and material at the EMT level PLUS the following material:

I. Routes of Administration
    A. Alimentary Tract
        1. Oral
        2. Sublingual
    B. Parenteral
        1. Subcutaneous
        2. Intramuscular
        3. Intravenous
        4. Intraosseous
        5. Inhalational

II. Administration of Medication to a Patient
    A. The "Rights" of Drug Administration
        1. Right patient – prescribed to patient
        2. Right medication – patient condition
        3. Right route – patient condition
        4. Right dose – prescribed to patient
        5. Right time – within expiration date
    B. Drug Dose Calculations
        1. System of weights and measures
        2. Drug calculations
            a. Desired dose
            b. Concentration on hand
            c. Volume on hand
        3. Calculate
            a. Volume based bolus
            b. IV drip rate
    C. Techniques of Medication Administration (Advantages, Disadvantages, Techniques)
        1. Peripheral venous cannulation
        2. Intraosseous

3. Intramuscular (manual)
4. Subcutaneous (manual)
5. Aerosolized
6. Nebulized
7. Sublingual
8. Intranasal

D. Reassessment
1. Data – Indications for medication
2. Action – Medication administered
3. Response – Effect of medication

E. Documentation

Pharmacology
Emergency Medications

AEMT Education Standard

Applies (to patient assessment and management) fundamental knowledge of the medications carried by AEMTs that may be administered to a patient during an emergency.

AEMT-Level Instructional Guideline

The AEMT Instructional Guidelines in this section include all the topics and material at the EMT level PLUS the following material:

The AEMT must know (to a fundamental depth) the names, mechanism of action, indications, contraindications, complications, routes of administration, side effects, interactions, dose, and any specific administration considerations, for all of the following emergency medications and intravenous fluids. Individual training programs have the authority to add any medication used locally by AEMTs.

I. Specific Medications
   A. Albuterol
   B. Aspirin
   C. Dextrose (50%)
   D. Epinephrine (Intramuscular or Subcutaneous)
   E. Glucagon
   F. Glucose
   G. Intravenous Fluids
      1. Dextrose 5% in water
      2. Normal Saline
      3. Lactated Ringer's
   H. Naloxone
   I. Nitroglycerin
      1. Paste
      2. Spray
      3. Tablets
   J. Oxygen
   K. Nitrous Oxide

II. Special Considerations in Pediatrics and Geriatrics
   A. Routes of Administration
   B. Dosages
   C. Dilutions
   D. Pharmacokinetic Alterations

Airway Management, Respiration, and Artificial Ventilation
Airway Management

AEMT Education Standard

Applies knowledge (fundamental depth, foundational breadth) of upper airway anatomy and physiology to patient assessment and management in order to assure a patent airway, adequate mechanical ventilation, and respiration for patients of all ages.

AEMT-Level Instructional Guideline

The AMT Instructional Guidelines in this section include all the topics and material at the EMT level PLUS the following material:

I.   Airway Anatomy
    A.   Sinuses
    B.   Upper Airway Tract
        1.   Nose
            a.   Warm and humidify air
            b.   Turbinate
        2.   Mouth and Oral Cavity
            a.   Lips
            b.   Teeth
            c.   Tongue
            d.   Soft Palate -- Uvula
            e.   Tonsils and Adenoids
        3.   Jaw
            a.   Facial Bones
                i.   maxilla
                ii.   mandible
        4.   Pharynx
            a.   Nasopharynx
            b.   Oropharynx
            c.   Hypopharynx
            d.   Laryngopharynx
        5.   Larynx
            a.   Cartilages
                i.   epiglottis
                ii.   arytenoid cartilages
                iii.   vocal cords
                iv.   thyroid cartilage
                v.   cricoid ring
            b.   Bone
    C.   Jugular Notch

D. Lower Airway Tract
　　1. Trachea
　　2. Carina
　　3. Bronchi
　　4. Lungs
　　　　a. Bronchioles
　　　　　　i. bronchial smooth muscle
　　　　　　ii. beta 2 adrenergic receptors
　　　　b. Pulmonary cilia
　　　　c. Alveoli
E. Support Structures
　　1. Chest Cage
　　　　a. Ribs
　　　　b. Muscles of respiration
　　　　　　i. intercostal muscles
　　　　　　ii. diaphragm
　　　　c. Pleura
　　　　　　i. parietal pleura
　　　　　　ii. visceral pleura
　　2. Phrenic nerve
　　3. Mediastinum

II. Airway Assessment
　A. Purpose
　　1. Identify inadequate airway
　　2. Identify an unstable airway
　　3. Identify potentially difficult airways
　B. Procedure
　　1. Gag Reflex
　　2. Airway obstruction
　　　　a. Soft tissue obstruction
　　　　b. Foreign bodies
　　　　c. Complete and incomplete
　　　　d. Upper vs. Lower
　　3. Work of breathing
　　4. Laryngospasm
　　5. Laryngeal edema
　　6. Penetrating injuries

III. Techniques of Assuring a Patent Airway
　A. Manual Airway Maneuvers
　B. Mechanical Airway Devices
　C. Relief of Foreign Body Airway Obstruction (Refer to Current American Heart Association Guidelines)

D.   Upper Airway Suctioning
1.   Review and elaborate on the upper airway suctioning material from the EMR and EMT levels
2.   Procedure for lower airway suctioning of the previously intubated patient
     a.   Purpose
     b.   Indications
     c.   Contraindications
     d.   Complications
     e.   Procedure
     f.   Limitation
E.   Blind Insertion Airway Devices
1.   Esophageal obturation (e.g., Combitube, PTL, Easytube, King LTD)
     a.   Purpose
     b.   Indications
     c.   Contraindications
     d.   Complications
     e.   Procedure (including confirmation techniques)
2.   Supraglottic devices (e.g., LMA, COBRA)
     a.   Purpose
     b.   Indications
     c.   Contraindications
     d.   Complications
     e.   Procedure (including confirmation techniques)

IV.   Consider Age-Related Variations in Pediatric and Geriatric Patients

Airway Management, Respiration, and Artificial Ventilation
Respiration

AEMT Education Standard

Applies knowledge (fundamental depth, foundational breadth) of upper airway anatomy and physiology to patient assessment and management in order to assure a patent airway, adequate mechanical ventilation, and respiration for patients of all ages.

AEMT-Level Instructional Guideline

The AMT Instructional Guidelines in this section include all the topics and material at the EMT level PLUS the following material:

I. Anatomy of the Respiratory System
    A. Includes All Airway Anatomy Covered in the Airway Management Section
    B. Additional Respiratory System Anatomy
    C. Chest Cage
        1. Ribs
        2. Muscles of respiration
            a. Intercostal muscles
            b. Diaphragm
        3. Pleura
            a. Parietal pleura
            b. Visceral pleura
    D. Phrenic Nerve
    E. Mediastinum

II. Physiology of Respiration
    A. Mechanics of Respiration
        1. Pulmonary ventilation
            a. Movement of the thoracic wall
            b. Intrathoracic pressure gradients
            c. Phases of ventilation
                i.   active phase
                ii. passive phase
            d. Lung volumes and capacities
                i.   volumes
                     a) tidal volume
                     b) minute volume
                     c) residual volume
                     d) dead space volume
                ii. capacities
                     a) vital capacity

                  iii.   maximum inspiratory force
                  iv.   maximum expiratory force
                  v.   significance of pulmonary volumes and capacities

      2.   Gas exchange
      3.   Oxygenation
      4.   Respiration
          a.   External
          b.   Internal
          c.   Cellular
      5.   Lung compliance

III.   Pathophysiology of Respiration
    A.   Pulmonary Ventilation
      1.   Interruption of nervous control
          a.   Drugs
          b.   Trauma
          c.   Muscular dystrophy
      2.   Structural damage to the thorax
      3.   Bronchoconstriction
      4.   Disruption of airway patency
          a.   Infection
          b.   Trauma/burns
          c.   Foreign body obstruction
          d.   Allergic reaction
          e.   Unconsciousness (loss of muscle tone)
    B.   Oxygenation
    C.   Respiration
      1.   External
          a.   Deficiencies due to altitude
          b.   Deficiencies due to closed environments
          c.   Deficiencies due to toxic or poisonous environments
      2.   Internal
          a.   Pathology typically related to changes in alveolar - capillary gas exchange
          b.   Typical disease processes
                i.   emphysema
                ii.   pulmonary edema
                iii.   pneumonia
                iv.   environmental/occupational exposure
                v.   drowning
      3.   Cellular

IV.   Assessment of Adequate and Inadequate Respiration

V.   Management of Adequate and Inadequate Respiration
      A.   Respiratory Compromise
            1.   Assure an adequate airway
            2.   Review supplemental oxygen therapy
            3.   Assisted positive pressure ventilations
                  a.   Purpose/definition
                  b.   Indications
                  c.   Contraindications
                  d.   Complications
                  e.   Procedure

VI.   Supplemental Oxygen Therapy
      A.   Review of Oxygen Delivery Devices Used by EMTs
            1.   Purpose
            2.   Indications
            3.   Contraindications
            4.   Complications
            5.   Procedures

VII. Age-Related Variations in Pediatric and Geriatric Patients

Artificial Ventilation

AEMT Education Standard

Applies knowledge (fundamental depth, foundational breadth) of upper airway anatomy and physiology to patient assessment and management in order to assure a patent airway, adequate mechanical ventilation, and respiration for patients of all ages.

AEMT-Level Instructional Guideline

The AMT Instructional Guidelines in this section include all the topics and material at the EMT level PLUS the following material:

I. Comprehensive Ventilation Assessment
  A. Purpose
  B. Procedure
  C. Minute Volume
  D. Alveolar Volume
  E. Evaluating the Effects of Artificial Ventilation
  F. Pulse Oximetry
    1. purpose
    2. Indications
    3. Contraindications
    4. Complications
    5. Procedure

II. The Management of Inadequate Ventilation
  A. Assure an Adequate Airway
  B. Supplemental Oxygen Therapy
  C. Artificial Ventilation Devices
    1. Bag-valve-mask with reservoir
      a. Advantages
      b. Disadvantages
    2. Manually triggered ventilation device
      a. Advantages
        i. allows a single rescuer to use both hands to maintain a mask-to-face seal while providing positive pressure ventilation to a patient.
        ii. reduces rescuer fatigue during extended transport times
      b. Disadvantages
        i. difficult to maintain adequate ventilation without assistance

    ii.   requires oxygen however, typical adult ventilation consumes 5 liters per minute o_2 versus 15 –25 liters per minute for a bag-valve-mask.
    iii.   typically used on adult patients only
    iv.   requires special unit and additional training for use in pediatric patients
    v.   the rescuer is unable to easily assess lung compliance.
    vi.   high ventilatory pressures may damage lung tissue.

3.   Automatic Transport Ventilator/Resuscitator
    a.   Advantages
    b.   Disadvantages
        i.   requires oxygen however, typical adult ventilation consumes 5 liters per minute 0_2 versus 15 –25 liters per minute for a bag-valve-mask.
        ii.   may require an external power source
        iii.   must have bag-valve-mask device available
        iv.   may interfere with timing of chest compressions during CPR
        v.   must monitor to assure full exhalation
        vi.   barotrauma

D.   Ventilation of an Apneic Patient
    1.   Purpose
    2.   Indications
    3.   Contraindications
    4.   Procedure

E.   Ventilation of the Protected Airway
    1.   Purpose
    2.   Indications
    3.   Contraindications
    4.   Complications
    5.   Procedure

III.   The Differences Between Normal and Positive Pressure Ventilation
    A.   Air Movement
        1.   Normal ventilation
            a.   Negative intrathoracic pressure
            b.   Air is sucked into lungs
        2.   Positive pressure ventilation
    B.   Blood Movement
        1.   Normal ventilation
            a.   Blood return from the body happens naturally
            b.   Blood is pulled back to the heart during normal breathing
        2.   Positive pressure ventilation
            a.   Venous return is decreased during lung inflation
            b.   Amount of blood pumped out of the heart is reduced.

C. Airway Wall Pressure
    1. Normal ventilation
    2. Positive pressure ventilation
        a. Walls are pushed out of normal anatomical shape
        b. More volume is required to have the same effect as normal breathing
D. Esophageal Opening Pressure
    1. Normal ventilation
    2. Positive pressure ventilation
        a. Air is pushed into the stomach during ventilation
        b. Gastric distention may lead to vomiting
E. Over Ventilation (Either by Rate or Volume) Can Be Detrimental to the Patient
    1. Hypotension
    2. Gastric distention
    3. Other unintended consequences

IV. Consider Age-Related Variations in Pediatric and Geriatric Patients

Patient Assessment
Scene Size-Up

Applies scene information and patient assessment findings (scene size-up, primary and secondary assessment, patient history, reassessment) to guide emergency management.

The AEMT Instructional Guidelines in this section include all the topics and material at the EMT level.

Patient Assessment
Primary Assessment

AEMT Education Standard

Applies scene information and patient assessment findings (scene size-up, primary and secondary assessment, patient history, reassessment) to guide emergency management.

AEMT-Level Instructional Guideline

The AEMT Instructional Guidelines in this section include all the topics and material at the EMT level PLUS the following material:

I. Primary Survey/Primary Assessment
    A. Initial General Impression - Based on The Patient's Age-Appropriate Appearance
        1. Appears stable
        2. Appears stable but potentially unstable
        3. Appears unstable
    B. Level of Consciousness
        1. Alert
        2. Responds to verbal stimuli.
        3. Responds to painful stimuli.
        4. Unresponsive - no gag or cough
    C. Airway Status
        1. Unresponsive patient
            a. Open the airway.
            b. Clear any obstructions
        2. Responsive patient - Is the patient talking or crying?
            a. If yes, assess for adequacy of breathing
            b. If no, open airway
    D. Breathing Status
        1. Patient responsive
            a. Breathing is adequate (rate and quality)
            b. Breathing is too fast (> 24 breaths per minute)
            c. Breathing is too slow (<8 breaths per minute)
            d. Breathing absent (choking)
        2. Patient unresponsive
            a. Breathing is adequate (rate and quality)
            b. Breathing is inadequate
            c. Breathing is absent
    E. Circulatory Status
        1. Radial pulse present (rate and quality)
            a. Normal rate
            b. Fast

              c.   Slow
              d.   Irregular rate

       2.   Radial pulse absent
       3.   Assess if major bleeding is present
       4.   Perfusion status
              a.   Skin color
              b.   Skin temperature
              c.   Skin moisture
              d.   Capillary refill (as appropriate)

F.   Identify Life Threats
G.   Assessment of Vital Functions

II.   Integration of Treatment/Procedures Needed to Preserve Life

III.   Evaluating Priority of Patient Care and Transport
      A.   Primary Assessment: Stable
      B.   Primary Assessment: Potentially Unstable
      C.   Primary Assessment: Unstable

Patient Assessment
History-Taking

AEMT Education Standard

Applies scene information and patient assessment findings (scene size-up, primary and secondary assessment, patient history, reassessment) to guide emergency management.

AEMT-Level Instructional Guideline

The AEMT Instructional Guidelines in this section include all the topics and material at the EMT level.

Patient Assessment
Secondary Assessment

AEMT Education Standard

Applies scene information and patient assessment findings (scene size-up, primary and secondary assessment, patient history, reassessment) to guide emergency management.

AEMT-Level Instructional Guideline

The AEMT Instructional Guidelines in this section include all the topics and material at the EMT level PLUS the following material:

I.   Assessment of Lung Sounds
    A.   Expose the Chest as Appropriate for the Environment
    B.   Auscultation
        1.   Technique
            a.   Medical versus trauma
            b.   Anterior chest
        2.   Lung sounds
            a.   Vesicular
            b.   Bronchovesicular
            c.   Bronchial sounds
            d.   Adventitious sounds
            e.   Absence of breath sounds
        3.   Inspiratory versus expiratory phase

II.   Special Considerations for Pediatric and Geriatric Patients
    A.   Normal Vital Signs by Age
    B.   See Special Patient Populations section

Patient Assessment
Monitoring Devices

AEMT Education Standard

Applies scene information and patient assessment findings (scene size-up, primary and secondary assessment, patient history, reassessment) to guide emergency management.

AEMT-Level Instructional Guideline

The AEMT Instructional Guidelines in this section include all the topics and material at the EMT level PLUS the following material:

I.   Blood Glucose Determination
    A.   Purpose
        1.   Assess blood glucose level
        2.   Assess impact of interventions
    B.   Indications
        1.   Decreased level of consciousness in the suspected diabetic
        2.   Decreased level of consciousness of unknown origin
    C.   Procedure
        1.   Cleaning the site
        2.   Refer to manufacturer's instructions for device being used
        3.   Disposal of sharps
    D.   Limitations
        1.   Lack of calibration
        2.   Venous versus Capillary sampling
    E.   Interpretation (see Medical Emergencies: Endocrine)

II.   Other Monitoring Devices
    A.   As additional monitoring devices become recognized as the "standard of care" in the out-of-hospital setting, those devices should be incorporated into the primary education of those who will be expected to use them in practice
    B.   State regulatory processes may elect to expand, delete, or modify from the monitor devices in this section

Patient Assessment
Reassessment

AEMT Education Standard

Applies scene information and patient assessment findings (scene size-up, primary and secondary assessment, patient history, reassessment) to guide emergency management.

AEMT-Level Instructional Guideline

The AEMT Instructional Guidelines in this section include all the topics and material at the EMT level.

Medicine
Medical Overview

AEMT Education Standard

Applies fundamental knowledge to provide basic and selected advanced emergency care and transportation based on assessment findings for an acutely ill patient.

AEMT-Level Instructional Guideline

The AEMT Instructional Guidelines in this section include all the topics and material at the EMT level PLUS the following material:

I.   Assessment Factors
    A.   Scene Safety
    B.   Environment
    C.   Chief Complaint
        1.   Primary reason for EMS response
        2.   Verbal or non-verbal
        3.   Possibly misleading
    D.   Life-Threatening Conditions
    E.   Non-Life-Threatening Conditions
    F.   Distracting Injuries
    G.   Tunnel Vision
    H.   Patient Cooperation
    I.   AEMT Attitude

II.   Major Components of the Patient Assessment
    A.   Standard Precautions
    B.   Scene Size-Up
    C.   General Impression
    D.   Initial Assessment
    E.   SAMPLE History
        1.   Importance of a thorough history
            a.   Primary component of the overall assessment of the medical patient
            b.   Requires a balance of knowledge and skill to obtain a thorough and accurate history
            c.   Helps to ensure the proper care will be provided for the patient.
        2.   Unresponsive patient
            a.   May be obtained from evidence at the scene
                i.   pill containers
                ii.   medical jewelry
            b.   May be obtained by family members or bystanders

3. Responsive patient
    a. obtained directly from the patient
    b. focused on the patient's chief complaint
    c. Additional history may be obtained from evidence at the scene
        i. pill containers
        ii. medical jewelry
        iii. family members
        iv. bystanders
4. OPQRST Mnemonic for evaluation of pain
    a. O – Onset
        i. focuses on what the patient was doing when the problem began.
        ii. question: what were you doing when the problem began?
    b. P – Provoke
        i. focuses on what might provoke the problem for the patient.
        ii. question: does anything you do make the problem better or worse?
    c. Q – Quality
        i. focuses on the patients own description of the problem.
        ii. questions
            a) can you describe your pain/discomfort?
            b) what does if feel like?
            c) is it sharp? dull?
            d) is it steady or does it come and go?
    d. R - Region/Radiate
        i. focuses on the specific area of the pain/discomfort.
        ii. questions
            a) can you point with one finger where you fee the pain/discomfort the most?
            b) does the pain/discomfort radiate to any other areas of your body?
    e. S – Severity
        i. focuses on the severity of the pain/discomfort.
        ii. questions
            a) on a scale of 1 to 10, with 10 being the worst pain you have ever felt, how would you rate your pain right now?
            b) how would you rate your pain when it first began?
            c) has there been any change since it first began?
    f. T – time
        i. focuses on the duration of the problem/pain/discomfort.
        ii. questions: when did your problem/pain/discomfort first begin?
F. Baseline Vital Signs

G. Secondary Assessment
1. May not be appropriate to perform a complete secondary assessment on all medical patients
2. Designed to identify any signs or symptoms of illness that may not have been revealed during the initial assessment.
   a. Head/scalp
      i. pain
      ii. symmetry
   b. Face
      i. pain
      ii. symmetry of facial muscles
   c. Eyes
      i. pupil size
      ii. equality and reactivity to light
      iii. pink moist conjunctiva
   d. Ears
      i. pain
      ii. drainage
   e. Nose
      i. pain
      ii. nasal flaring
   f. Mouth
      i. foreign body
      ii. loose dentures
      iii. pink & moist mucosa
   g. Neck
      i. pain
      ii. accessory muscle use
      iii. jugular vein distention
      iv. medical jewelry
      v. stoma
   h. Chest
      i. pain
      ii. equal rise and fall
      iii. guarding
      iv. breath sounds
      v. retractions
      vi. scars
   i. Abdomen
      i. pain
      ii. rigidity
      iii. distention
      iv. scars
   j. Pelvis/genital
      i. pain
      ii. incontinence

            k.   Arms
                  i.   pain
                  ii.   distal circulation
                  iii.   sensation
                  iv.   motor function
                  v.   track marks
                  vi.   medical jewelry
            l.   Legs
                  i.   pain
                  ii.   distal circulation
                  iii.   sensation
                  iv.   motor function
                  v.   track marks
                  vi.   medical jewelry
            m.   Back
                  i.   pain
                  ii.   scars
H.   Continued Assessment
      1.   When practical, transport the patient in the recovery position to help
            ensure a patent airway
      2.   Consider the need for ALS backup

Medicine
Neurology

AEMT Education Standard

Applies fundamental knowledge to provide basic and selected advanced emergency care and transportation based on assessment findings for an acutely ill patient.

AEMT-Level Instructional Guideline

The AEMT Instructional Guidelines in this section include all the topics and material at the EMT level PLUS the following material:

I. Stroke/TIA
    A. Causes
        1. Hemorrhage
        2. Clot
    B. Review of Anatomy and Function of the Brain and Cerebral Blood Vessels
    C. Assessment Findings and Symptoms
        1. Confused, dizzy, weak
        2. Decreasing or increasing level of consciousness
        3. Combative or uncooperative or restless
        4. Facial drooping, inability to swallow, tongue deviation
        5. Double vision or blurred vision
        6. Difficulty speaking or absence speech
        7. Decreased or absent movement of one or more extremities
        8. Headache
        9. Decreased or absent sensation in one or more extremities or other areas of body
        10. Coma
    D. Stroke Alert Criteria
        1. Cincinnati Prehospital Stroke Scale
        2. Other stroke scales
    E. Management of Patient With Stroke Assessment Findings or Symptoms
    F. Scene Safety and Standard Precautions
        1. ABCs /position
        2. Oxygen/suction
        3. Pulse oximetry
        4. Emotional support
        5. Rapid transport
    G. Transient Ischemic Attack (TIA)

II. Seizures
    A. Incidence
    B. Caused by Hypoglycemia
        1. Pathophysiology
        2. Assessment
        3. Management
    C. Types of Seizures
        1. Generalized tonic-clonic
            a. Aura
            b. Tonic
            c. Clonic
            d. Postictal
        2. Partial seizures
        3. Status epilepticus
    D. Assessment Findings
        1. Spasms, muscle contractions
        2. Bite tongue, increased secretions
        3. Sweating
        4. Cyanosis
        5. Unconscious gradually increasing level of consciousness
        6. May shaking or tremors and no loss of consciousness
        7. Incontinent
        8. Amnesia of event
    E. Management
        1. Safety of patient/position
        2. ABCs, consider nasopharyngeal airway
        3. Oxygen/suction
        4. Pulse oximetry
        5. Emotional support

III. Headache
    A. As a Symptom
    B. As a Neurological Condition
    C. Assessment Findings and Symptoms
    D. Management

IV. Age-Related Variations for Pediatric and Geriatric Assessment and Management
    A. Pediatrics
        1. Epidemiology
        2. Anatomic and physiologic differences in children
        3. Pathophysiology
        4. Causes of altered mental status in children
        5. Assessment
            a. History
            b. Physical findings
        6. Meningitis

          7.   Seizures
          8.   Altered mental status
          9.   Management
    B.   Geriatrics - Stroke Common in This Age Group

V.   Communication and Documentation

VI.   Transport Decisions—Rapid Transport to Appropriate Facility

Medicine
Abdominal and Gastrointestinal Disorders

AEMT Education Standard

Applies fundamental knowledge to provide basic and selected advanced emergency care and transportation based on assessment findings for an acutely ill patient.

AEMT-Level Instructional Guideline

The AEMT Instructional Guidelines in this section include all the topics and material at the EMT level PLUS the following material:

I.   Define Acute Abdomen

II.   Anatomy of the Organs of the Abdominopelvic Cavity
    A.   Stomach
    B.   Intestines
    C.   Esophagus
    D.   Spleen
    E.   Urinary Bladder
    F.   Liver
    G.   Gall Bladder
    H.   Pancreas
    I.   Kidney
    J.   Reproductive Organs

III. Assessment and Symptoms
    A.   Techniques
        1.   Inspection
        2.   Palpation
    B.   Normal Findings—Soft Non-Tender
    C.   Abnormal Findings
        1.   Nausea/vomiting
            a.   Excessive
            b.   Hematemesis
        2.   Change in bowel habits/stool
            a.   Constipation
            b.   Diarrhea
            c.   Dark tarry stool
        3.   Urination
            a.   Pain
            b.   Frequency

         c.   Color
         d.   Odor
    4.   Weight loss
    5.   Belching/flatulence
    6.   Concurrent chest pain
    7.   Pain, tenderness, guarding, distension
    8.   Other

IV.   General Management for Patients With an Acute Abdomen
    A.   Scene Safety and Standard Precautions
    B.   Airway, Ventilatory and Circulation
    C.   Position
    D.   Emotional Support

V.   Specific Acute Abdominal Conditions—Definition, Causes, Assessment Findings and Symptoms, Complications, and Specific Prehospital Management.
    A.   Acute and Chronic Gastrointestinal Hemorrhage
    B.   Peritonitis
    C.   Ulcerative Diseases

VI.   Consider Age-Related Variations for Pediatric and Geriatric Assessment and Management

VII.   Pediatrics
    A.   Anatomic and Physiologic Differences in Children
    B.   Pathophysiology
    C.   Assessment
        1.   History
        2.   Physical findings
            a.   Vomiting causes dehydration
            b.   Appendicitis common in children
            c.   Abdominal pain from constipation
            d.   Vomiting
            e.   GI Bleeding
        3.   Management
    D.   Geriatric
        1.   May not exhibit rigidity or guarding
        2.   Abdominal pain related to cardiac conditions

VIII.   Communication and Documentation for Patients With an Abdominal or Gastrointestinal Condition or Emergency

IX.   Transport Decisions

Medicine
Immunology

AEMT Education Standard

Applies fundamental knowledge to provide basic and selected advanced emergency care and transportation based on assessment findings for an acutely ill patient.

AEMT-Level Instructional Guideline

The AEMT Instructional Guidelines in this section include all the topics and material at the EMT level PLUS the following material:

I.   Introduction
     A.   Definition of Terms
          1.   Allergic reaction
          2.   Anaphylaxis
     B.   Risk Factors and Common Allergens

II.   Basic Immune System's Response to Allergens
     A.   The Purpose of the Response
     B.   The Type of Response (Local versus Systemic)
     C.   The Speed of the Response

III.   Pathophysiology
     A.   Allergic Reaction
          1.   Antigens
          2.   Antibodies
          3.   Mast cells and basophils
          4.   Histamine, leukotrienes, and other mediators
          5.   Local reactions
          6.   Reactions

IV.   Assessment
     A.   Mild Allergic Reaction
          1.   Cutaneous
          2.   Other
     B.   Moderate Allergic Reaction
          1.   Upper airway
          2.   Lower airway
          3.   Cardiovascular
          4.   Cutaneous
          5.   Gastrointestinal
          6.   Neurological

C. Severe Allergic Reaction/Anaphylaxis
1. Upper airway
2. Lower airway
3. Cardiovascular
4. Cutaneous
5. Gastrointestinal
6. Neurological

V. Managing Anaphylaxis
A. Provide Treatment Specific to Assessment Findings and Severity of Reaction
B. Remove Allergen If Possible
C. Protect the Airway
D. Oxygenate the Patient
E. Ventilate If Needed
1. Apneic patient
2. Dyspneic patient
3. Patient with airway edema
F. Medication Administration
1. Epinephrine administration
2. Bronchodilation
G. Fluid Administration

VI. Age-Related Considerations
A. Pediatric Epinephrine Dosing
B. Use of Epinephrine in the Geriatric Patient

Medicine
Infectious Disease

AEMT Education Standard

Applies fundamental knowledge to provide basic and selected advanced emergency care and transportation based on assessment findings for an acutely ill patient.

AEMT-Level Instructional Guideline

The AEMT Instructional Guidelines in this section include all the topics and material at the EMT level PLUS the following material:

I.   Causes of Infectious Disease
     A.   Infectious Agents
          1.   Bacteria
          2.   Viruses
          3.   Fungi
          4.   Protozoa
          5.   Helminths (worms)

II.   Standard Precautions, Personal Protective Equipment, and Cleaning and Disposing of Equipment and Supplies
     A.   Principles of Standard Precautions
     B.   Hand Washing Guidelines
     C.   Recommendations for Personal Protective Equipment
     D.   Recommendations for Cleaning or Sterilization of Equipment
     E.   Recommendations for Disposing of Contaminated Linens and Supplies Including Sharps
     F.   Recommendations for Decontaminating the Ambulance

III.   Specific Diseases and Conditions
     A.   HIV and AIDS
          1.   Incidence, morbidity, mortality, risk factors, modes of transmission
          2.   Pathophysiology
          3.   Body systems affected
          4.   Progression of disease including opportunistic infections
          5.   Healthcare worker susceptibility and transmission
          6.   Assessment findings and symptoms
               a.   Often asymptomatic
               b.   Non-specific febrile illness
               c.   Sore throat, fatigue
               d.   Swollen spleen and lymph glands

   e. Weight loss

   f. Opportunistic infections

  7. Management for a patient with HIV or AIDS-related conditions

   a. Prehospital care is supportive

   b. Manage airway and support ventilation

   c. IV if needed

   d. Respiratory isolation if coughing

  8. Immunization and treatment of exposure

 B. Hepatitis

  1. Introduction--Pathophysiology, incidence, types, causes, risk factors, methods of transmission, complications

  2. General assessment findings and symptoms

   a. Asymptomatic

   b. Non-specific febrile illness

   c. Light-colored stools

   d. Dark urine

   e. Fatigue

   f. Nausea/vomiting

   g. Abdominal pain/tenderness

   h. Jaundice

   i. Fulminant acute hepatitis

  3. Treatments for exposure/prevention; immunizations

  4. Types

   a. Hepatitis A

   b. Hepatitis B

   c. Hepatitis C

   d. Hepatitis D

   e. Hepatitis E

   f. Hepatitis G

   g. Other

  5. Management for a patient with hepatitis

   a. Prehospital care is supportive

   b. Manage airway and support ventilation

   c. IV if needed

IV. Consider Age-Related Variations in Pediatric and Geriatric Patients as They Relate Assessment and Managements of Patients With a Gastrointestinal Condition or Emergency

V. Communication and Documentation for a Patient With a Communicable or Infectious Disease

VI. Transport Decisions Including Special Infection Control Procedures

VII. Legal Requirements Regarding Reporting Communicable or Infectious Diseases/Conditions
    A. Exposure of Health Care Provider
        1. Current recommended treatment modalities and follow up
        2. Prevention of exposure or immunizations/vaccines
    B. Required Reporting to the Health Department or Other Heath Care Agency

Medicine
Endocrine Disorders

Applies fundamental knowledge to provide basic and selected advanced emergency care and transportation based on assessment findings for an acutely ill patient.

AEMT-Level Instructional Guideline

The AEMT Instructional Guidelines in this section include all the topics and material at the EMT level PLUS the following material:

I.   Diabetic Emergencies
    A.   Related Anatomy of the Pancreas and Organs Supporting Blood Sugar Regulation
    B.   Physiology of the Pancreas
    C.   Hormones Related to Blood Sugar Regulation
    D.   Pathophysiology of Diabetes Mellitus
        1.   Long-term complications
        2.   Types of diabetes
            a.   Type I
            b.   Type II
            c.   Gestational
    E.   Drugs to Manage Diabetes
        1.   Insulins
            a.   types
            b.   delivery methods
        2.   Oral antihyperglycemics

II.   Assessment
    A.   Impact of Disease on Prehospital Assessment
    B.   Alterations of Findings in Long-Term Diabetics
    C.   Hypoglycemia
        1.   Physical findings
        2.   Blood sugar level
        3.   Causes
    D.   Hyperglycemia/DKA
        1.   Physical findings
        2.   Blood sugar level
        3.   Causes
    E.   Treatment
        1.   Oxygenation and ventilation requirements
        2.   Blood glucose determination
        3.   Oral glucose

4. Glucagon administration
5. IV placement and fluid therapy for
   a. hyperglycemia
   b. hypoglycemia
6. D50 Administration
F. Reassessment and Evaluation for Other Underlying Acute Illness in the Hyperglycemic Patient

III. Age-Related Considerations
1. Pediatric patients
2. Usually type I diabetes
3. Late stages of hyperglycemia may have cerebral edema
4. Prone to seizures
5. Prone to dehydration in hyperglycemia
6. Geriatric patients
7. Masking of illness through changes in pain perception
8. Prone to dehydration and sepsis

IV. Communication and Documentation

Medicine
Psychiatric

AEMT Education Standard

Applies fundamental knowledge to provide basic and selected advanced emergency care and transportation based on assessment findings for an acutely ill patient.

AEMT-Level Instructional Guideline

The AEMT Instructional Guidelines in this section include all the topics and material at the EMT level PLUS the following material:

I.   Define
    A.   Behavior
    B.   Psychiatric Disorder
    C.   Behavioral Emergency

II.   Epidemiology of Psychiatric Disorders

III.   Assessment
    A.   General Appearance
    B.   Speech
    C.   Skin
    D.   Posture/Gait
    E.   Mental Status
    F.   Mood, Thought, Perception, Judgment, Memory, and Attention

IV.   Behavioral Change
    A.   Factors That May Alter a Patient's Behavior – May Include Situational Stresses, Medical Illnesses, Psychiatric Problems, and Alcohol Or Drugs
    B.   Common Causes of Behavioral Alteration
        1.   Low blood sugar
        2.   Lack of oxygen
        3.   Hypoperfusion
        4.   Head trauma
        5.   Mind altering substances
        6.   Psychogenic – resulting in psychotic thinking, depression or panic
        7.   Excessive cold
        8.   Excessive heat
        9.   Meningitis
        10.   Seizure disorders
        11.   Toxic ingestions—overdose
        12.   Withdrawal of drugs or alcohol

V. Psychiatric Emergencies
- A. Acute Psychosis
  - 1. Assessment for Suicide Risk
    - a. Depression
    - b. Risk Factors/signs or symptoms
      - i. ideation or defined lethal plan of action which has been verbalized and/or written.
      - ii. alcohol and substance abuse
      - iii. purposelessness
      - iv. anxiety, agitation, unable to sleep or sleeping all the time
      - v. feeling trapped, no way out
      - vi. hopelessness
      - vii. withdrawal from friends, family and society
      - viii. anger and/or aggressive tendencies
      - ix. recklessness or engaging in risky activities
      - x. dramatic mood changes
      - xi. history of trauma or abuse
      - xii. some major physical illness (cancer, CHF, etc.)
      - xiii. previous suicide attempt
      - xiv. job or financial loss
      - xv. relational or social loss
      - xvi. easy access to lethal means
      - xvii. lack of social support and sense of isolation
      - xviii. certain cultural and religious beliefs
  - 2. Important questions
    - a. How does the patient feel?
    - b. Determine suicidal tendencies
    - c. Is patient threat to self or others?
    - d. Is there a medical problem?
    - e. Is there trauma involved?
    - f. Interventions?
- B. Agitated Delirium
  - 1. Emergency medical care
    - a. Scene size-up, personal safety
    - b. Establish rapport
      - i. utilize therapeutic interviewing techniques
        - a) engage in active listening
        - b) supportive and empathetic
        - c) limit interruptions
        - d) respect patient's territory, limit physical touch
      - ii. avoid threatening actions, statements and questions
      - iii. approach slowly and purposefully
    - c. Patient assessment
      - i. intellectual functioning
      - ii. orientation
      - iii. memory

          iv.   concentration

          v.   judgment

          vi.   thought content

               a)   disordered thoughts

               b)   delusions, hallucinations

               c)   unusual worries, fears

          vii.   language

               a)   speech pattern and content

               b)   garbled or unintelligible

          viii.   mood

               a)   anxiety, depression, elation, agitation

               b)   level of alertness, distractibility

                     i)   appearance, hygiene, dress

                     ii)   psychomotor activity

    d.   Calm the patient – do not leave the patient alone, unless unsafe situation; consider need for law enforcement

    e.   Restrain if necessary

    f.   Transport

    g.   If overdose, bring medications or drugs found to medical facility.

VI.   Medical-Legal Considerations
    A.   Types of Restraints
    B.   Transport Against Patient Will

VII.   Consider Age-Related Variations for Pediatric and Geriatric Assessment and Management
    A.   Pediatric Behavioral Emergencies
         1.   Teenage suicide concerns
         2.   Aggressive behavior may be a symptom of an underlying disorder or disability
    B.   Geriatrics

Medicine
Cardiovascular

AEMT Education Standard

Applies fundamental knowledge to provide basic and selected advanced emergency care and transportation based on assessment findings for an acutely ill patient.

AEMT-Level Instructional Guideline

The AEMT Instructional Guidelines in this section include all the topics and material at the EMT level PLUS the following material:

I.   Anatomy of the Cardiovascular System
    A.   Location
        1.   Layers
            a.   Myocardium
            b.   Endocardium
            c.   Pericardium
                i.   visceral (epicardium)
                ii.   parietal
                iii.   pericardial fluid
        2.   Chambers
            a.   Atria
            b.   Ventricles
        3.   Valves
            a.   Atrioventricular (AV) valves
                i.   tricuspid (right)
                ii.   mitral (left)
            b.   Semilunar valves
                i.   pulmonic (right)
                ii.   aortic (left)
        4.   Myocardial blood supply
            a.   Arteries
            b.   Veins
        5.   Electrical and conduction system
            a.   Myocardial muscle cells
            b.   Specialized electrical cells
            c.   Automaticity
            d.   Autonomic Control
                i.   sympathetic
                ii.   parasympathetic
    B.   Vessels
        1.   Aorta

        2.   Arteries
        3.   Arterioles
        4.   Capillaries
        5.   Venules
        6.   Veins
        7.   Vena cava
   C.   Blood
        1.   Red blood cells
        2.   White blood cells
        3.   Platelets
        4.   Plasma

II.   Physiology
   A.   Cardiac Cycle
        1.   Systole
        2.   Diastole
   B.   Pulses
        1.   Peripheral pulses
        2.   Central pulses
   C.   Blood Pressure
        1.   Systolic
        2.   Diastolic
   D.   Blood Circulation Through a Double Pump
        1.   Respiratory system
            a.   Deoxygenated blood to lungs
            b.   Oxygenated blood back to heart
        2.   Body
   E.   Cardiac Output
   F.   Perfusion
        1.   Function of red blood cells in oxygen delivery
        2.   Factors governing adequate perfusion
            a.   Rate
            b.   Pump
            c.   Volume
   G.   Oxygenation of Tissues
        1.   Delivery of oxygenated blood
        2.   Removal of tissue wastes

III.   Angina Pectoris/Acute Coronary Syndrome
   A.   Epidemiology
   B.   Precipitating Causes
        1.   Atherosclerosis
        2.   Vasospastic (Prinzmetal's)
   C.   Morbidity/ Mortality
        1.   Not a self-limiting disease
        2.   Chest pain may dissipate, but myocardial ischemia and injury can continue

3.   A single anginal episode may be a precursor to myocardial infarction
4.   May not be cardiac in origin
5.   Must be diagnosed by a physician
6.   Related terminology
       a.   Defined as a brief discomfort, has predictable characteristics and is relieved promptly - no change in this pattern
       b.   Stable
           i.   occurs at a relative fixed frequency
           ii.   usually relieved by rest and/ or medication
       c.   Unstable
           i.   occurs without fixed frequency
           ii.   may or may not be relieved by rest and/ or medication
       d.   Initial - first episode
       e.   Progressive - accelerating in frequency and duration
       f.   Preinfarction angina
           i.   pain at rest
           ii.   sitting or lying down

D.   Primary Survey Findings
1.   Airway/ breathing
       a.   Labored breathing may or may not be present
2.   Circulation
       a.   Peripheral pulses
           i.   quality
           ii.   rhythm
       b.   Peripheral perfusion
           i.   changes in skin color
           ii.   changes in skin temperature
           iii.   changes in skin moisture

E.   History of the Present Illness/Sample History
1.   Chief complaint
       a.   Typical - sudden onset of discomfort, usually of brief duration, lasting three to five minutes, maybe five to 15 minutes; never 30 minutes to 2 hours
       b.   Typical - usually relieved by rest and/ or medication
       c.   Epigastric pain or discomfort
       d.   Atypical
2.   Denial
3.   Contributing history
       a.   Initial recognized event
       b.   Recurrent event
       c.   Increasing frequency and/or duration of event

F.   Secondary Survey Findings
1.   Airway
2.   Breathing
       a.   May or may not be labored
       b.   Breath sounds

              i.   may be clear to auscultation
              ii.   may be congested in the bases
        3.   Circulation
              a.   Alterations in heart rate and rhythm may occur
              b.   Peripheral pulses are usually not affected
              c.   Blood pressure may be elevated during the episode and normalize
                     afterwards
    G.   Management
        1.   Refer to American Heart Association guidelines
        2.   Rapid transport
              a.   Sense of urgency for reperfusion
              b.   No relief with medications
              c.   Hypotension/ hypoperfusion with CNS involvement

IV.   Acute Myocardial Infarction
    A.   Epidemiology
    B.   Precipitating Causes (as With Angina)
        1.   Atherosclerosis
        2.   Persistent angina
        3.   Occlusion
        4.   Non-traumatic
        5.   Trauma
    C.   Morbidity/Mortality
        1.   Sudden death
        2.   Extensive myocardial damage
        3.   May result in ventricular fibrillation
    D.   Primary Survey Findings
        1.   Airway/breathing
        2.   Circulation
              a.   Peripheral pulses
                     i.   quality
                     ii.   rhythm
              b.   Peripheral perfusion
                     i.   changes in skin color
                     ii.   changes in skim temperature
                     iii.   changes in skin moisture
    E.   History of the Present Illness/Sample History
        1.   Chief complaint
              a.   Typical onset of discomfort, usually of long duration, over 30
                     minutes
              b.   Typically unrelieved by rest and/ or nitroglycerin preparation
              c.   Epigastric pain or discomfort
              d.   Atypical
        2.   Contributing history
              a.   First time
              b.   Recurrent

   c. Increasing frequency and/ or duration

  3. Denial

F. Secondary Survey Findings

  1. Airway

  2. Breath sounds

   a. May be clear to auscultation

   b. Congestion in bases may be present

  3. Circulation

   a. Skin

    i. pallor during the episode

    ii. temperature may vary

    iii. diaphoresis is usually present

   b. Alterations in heart rate and rhythm may occur

   c. Peripheral pulses are usually not affected

   d. Blood pressure may be elevated or lowered

G. Management

  1. Refer to American Heart Association guidelines

   a. Scope of practice includes

    i. oxygen

    ii. aspirin

    iii. nitroglycerin

    iv. nitrous oxide

  2. Transport

   a. Criteria for rapid transport

    i. no relief with medications

    ii. hypotension/ hypoperfusion

V. Irregularity of Pulse

Medicine
Toxicology

AEMT Education Standard

Applies fundamental knowledge to provide basic and selected advanced emergency care and transportation based on assessment findings for an acutely ill patient.

AEMT-Level Instructional Guideline

The AEMT Instructional Guidelines in this section include all the topics and material at the EMT level PLUS the following material:

I.   Introduction
    A.   Define Toxicology, Poisoning, Overdose
    B.   National Poison Control Center
    C.   Routes of Absorption
        1.   Ingestion
        2.   Inhalation
        3.   Injection
        4.   Absorption

II.   Poisoning by Ingestion
    A.   Examples
    B.   Assessment Findings
    C.   General Management Considerations

III. Poisoning by Inhalation
    A.   Examples
    B.   Assessment Findings
    C.   General Management Considerations

IV.   Poisoning by Injection
    A.   Examples
    B.   Assessment Findings
    C.   General Management Considerations

V.   Poisoning by Absorption
    A.   Examples
    B.   Assessment Findings
    C.   General Management Considerations

VI. Drugs of Abuse
    A. Opiates/Narcotics
        1. Common causative agents
        2. Assessment findings and symptoms
            a. Decreased level of consciousness, sedation
            b. Hypotension
            c. Respiratory depression/ arrest
            d. Nausea, Pinpoint pupils
            e. Seizures and Coma
        3. Management for a patient using opiates
    B. Alcohol
        1. Overview of alcoholism including long term effects
        2. Alcohol abuse
            a. CNS changes—agitation to sedation to altered level of consciousness
            b. Respiratory depression
            c. Nausea and vomiting
            d. Uncoordination
        3. Alcohol withdrawal
            a. Tremors, sweating, weakness
            b. Hallucinations and seizures
        4. Assessment findings and symptoms for patients with alcohol abuse and alcohol withdrawal
        5. Management for a patient using alcohol or withdrawing from alcohol
    C. Common Causative Agents, Assessment Findings and Symptoms, Management
        1. Cannabis
        2. Hallucinogens
        3. Stimulants
        4. Barbiturates/sedatives/ hypnotics

VII. Poisonings and Exposures
    A. Scene Safety Issues
    B. Common causative agents, assessment findings and symptoms, management
        1. Pesticides
        2. Chemicals
        3. Household Cleaning poisonings
        4. Poisonous Plants

VIII. Medication Overdose
    A. Common Causes of Overdoses (Other Than Drugs of Abuse)
        1. Cardiac medications
        2. Psychiatric medications
        3. Non-prescription pain medications including Salicylates and Acetaminophen
        4. Other

B.   Assessment Findings and Symptoms for Patients With Medication Overdose
C.   Management for a Patient With Medication Overdose

IX.   General Treatment Modalities for Poisonings
      A.   Scene Safety
      B.   Standard Precautions and Decontamination
      C.   Airway Control
      D.   Ventilation and Oxygenation
      E.   Circulation
      F.   Use of Activated Charcoal
           1.   Indications/contraindications/side effects
           2.   Physician order
           3.   Dose

X.   Toxic Syndromes
      A.   Introduction
           1.   Definition of a toxic syndrome (toxidrome)
           2.   Incidence of opiate abuse
      B.   Opiate Intoxication/Poisoning
           1.   Common causative agents
                a.   heroin, morphine, methadone
                b.   codeine, meperidine, propoxyphene
                c.   fentanyl, lortab, oxycontin
                d.   other
           2.   Assessment findings specific to opiate intoxication/poisoning
                a.   CNS -- Level of consciousness/behavior
                    i.   euphoria
                    ii.   decreased level of consciousness
                    iii.   sedation
                    iv.   pin-point pupils
                    v.   seizures
                    vi.   coma
                b.   Respiratory
                    i.   decreased respiratory rate and effort
                    ii.   apnea
                c.   Gastrointestinal
                    i.   nausea
                    ii.   vomiting
           3.   Management specific to opiate intoxication/poisoning
                a.   Airway/Breathing support
                    i.   oxygenation requirements
                    ii.   ventilatory requirements
                          a)   considerations in use of oral pharyngeal airways
                        b)   bag-valve mask
                          c)   considerations of use of the advanced airway in the opiate overdose patient

        b.   Circulatory Support
             i.   causes of hypotension in the opiate overdose
             ii.   IV access
        c.   Pharmaceutical interventions
        d.   Other considerations in the care of the opiate overdose
             i.   underlying chronic illness
                   a)   HIV/AIDS
                   b)   hepatitis
                   c)   malnutrition
                   d)   sepsis
             ii.   family interaction and social issues
             iii.   chronic pain patients
                   a)   drug dependency
                   b)   consequences of narcotic antagonist use in the chronic pain patient

XI.   Consider Age-Related Variations for Pediatric and Geriatric Assessment and Management
      A.   Pediatric
          1.   Toddler-age prone to ingestions of toxic substance
          2.   Adolescent prone to experimentation with drugs of abuse
      B.   Geriatric
          1.   Alcoholism is common in elderly
          2.   drug dependency
          3.   consequences of narcotic antagonist use in the chronic pain patient

XII.   Documentation and Communication
      A.   Documentation of the Opiate Overdose Specific Patient
      B.   Communication
          1.   Hospital personnel
          2.   Family
          3.   Law enforcement personnel
      C.   Transport Decisions

Medicine
Respiratory

Applies fundamental knowledge to provide basic and selected advanced emergency care and transportation based on assessment findings for an acutely ill patient.

The AEMT Instructional Guidelines in this section include all the topics and material at the EMT level PLUS the following material:

I. Anatomy and Physiology
    A. Anatomy of the Pulmonary System
        1. Upper airway
            a. Function
            b. Structures and functions of:
                i.   nose and nasopharynx
                ii. pharynx
                iii. hypopharynx
                iv. larynx
        2. Lower airway
            a. Function
            b. Structures and functions of:
                i.   trachea
                ii. bronchi
                iii. bronchioles
                iv. cilia
        3. Gas exchange
            a. Function
            b. Structures and functions of;
                i.   alveoli
                ii. interstitial space
                iii. pulmonary capillary bed
        4. Chest wall
            a. Function
            b. Structures and function of:
                i.   diaphragm
                ii. intercostal muscles
                iii. accessory muscles
                iv. pleural space

5.   Neurological control of breathing
        a.   Function
        b.   Structures and functions:
            i.   medulla
            ii.   phrenic nerve
            iii.   spinal nerves
            iv.   Hering-Breuer reflex

II.   Pathophysiology
    A.   Obstructive/Restrictive Lung Diseases
        1.   Emphysema
            a.   changes in respiratory tract
            b.   changes in gas exchange
            c.   long term effects
            d.   decompensated states
        2.   Chronic Bronchitis
            a.   changes in respiratory tract
            b.   changes in gas exchange
            c.   long term effects
            d.   decompensated states
        3.   Asthma
            a.   changes in respiratory tract
            b.   changes in gas exchange
            c.   long term effects
            d.   decompensated states
    B.   Infectious Lung Disease
        1.   Pneumonia

III.   Assessment
    A.   Impact of Disease on Prehospital Assessment
        1.   Pertinent historical questions
        2.   Pertinent physical findings
            a.   Breath sounds
               i.   course crackles
               ii.   fine crackles
               iii.   ronchi
               iv.   wheezes
                  a)   diffuse
                  b)   continuous
               v.   stridor
               vi.   pleural rub
            b.   Inspiratory vs. Expiratory ratios
    B.   Finding Associated With Specific Diseases
        1.   Emphysema
        2.   Chronic Bronchitis
        3.   Asthma
        4.   Pneumonia

C.   Age-Related Considerations
     1.   Pediatrics
         a.   variations in symptomatology
         b.   variations in physical presentation
            i.   asthma
           ii.   types of pneumonia
     2.   Geriatrics
         a.   variations in symptomatology
         b.   variations in physical presentation

IV.   Treatment
     A.   Oxygenation and Ventilation Requirements
     B.   Use of Inhaled Beta-Agonists
     C.   IV Fluid Therapy in Respiratory Illness
     D.   Age-Related Considerations
        1.   Pediatrics
           a.   dosage considerations
           b.   fluid considerations
        2.   Geriatrics
           a.   drug interaction considerations
           b.   fluid considerations

V.   Communication and documentation

Medicine
Hematology

Applies fundamental knowledge to provide basic and selected advanced emergency care and transportation based on assessment findings for an acutely ill patient.

AEMT-Level Instructional Guideline

The AEMT Instructional Guidelines in this section include all the topics and material at the EMT level PLUS the following material:

I.   Introduction
     A.   Epidemiology of Blood Disorders
          1.   Incidence
          2.   Morbidity/mortality
     B.   Anatomy And Physiology
          1.   Blood
          2.   Plasma
          3.   Blood forming organs
          4.   Normal red cell production, function, destruction

II.   Sickle Cell Disease
     A.   Definition, Pathophysiology, Epidemiology, Mortality and Morbidity
          1.   Types of emergent presentations
               a.   Vaso-occlusive crisis
                    i.   description
                    ii.   signs and symptoms
                    iii.   implications
               b.   Acute chest syndrome
                    i.   description
                    ii.   signs and symptoms
                    iii.   implications
               c.   Acute splenic sequestration syndrome (pediatric)
                    i.   description
                    ii.   signs and symptoms
                    iii.   implications
          2.   Patient management
               a.   Administer high-concentration oxygen
               b.   Initiate IV therapy
               c.   Maintain normothermic
                d.   Rest
               e.   Pain management

III.   Assessment
     A.   Types of Presentation
     B.   Specific Signs and Symptoms

IV.   Management
     A.   Airway and Oxygenation Requirements
     B.   IV Access

V.   Age-Related Considerations
     A.   Types of Crisis Specific to the Pediatric Patient
     B.   Special Considerations in Treatment

VI.   Documentation and Communication

Medicine
Genitourinary/Renal

Applies fundamental knowledge to provide basic and selected advanced emergency care and transportation based on assessment findings for an acutely ill patient.

The AEMT Instructional Guidelines in this section include all the topics and material at the EMT level PLUS the following material:

I. Anatomy and Physiology
    A. Urinary System
        1. Structures
        2. Functions
    B. Pathophysiology
        1. Renal Calculi (kidney stones)
            a. Calculi formation
            b. Consequences of renal calculi
        2. Types of renal failure
            a. Acute
            b. Chronic
        3. End-stage renal disease
            a. Definition
            b. Causes
    C. Dialysis
        1. Definition of dialysis
        2. Process of dialysis
        3. Types of dialysis
        4. Complications/adverse effects of dialysis
            a. Hypotension
            b. Muscle cramps
            c. Nausea/vomiting
            d. Altered mentation, loss of consciousness
            e. Hemorrhage from shunt
            f. Air embolism
            g. Myocardial ischemia
            h. Infection
            i. Electrolyte imbalance
        5. Consequences of missed dialysis treatment
            a. Electrolyte excesses

        b.   Weakness

        c.   Pulmonary edema

D.   Assessment

    1.   Findings in renal calculi

    2.   Findings in renal failure

        a.   Acute

        b.   Chronic

        c.   End-stage

E.   Management

    1.   Renal calculi patient

        a.   Oxygen requirements

        b.   IV access

        c.   Fluid administration considerations

    2.   Renal failure patients

        a.   Oxygen and ventilation requirements

        b.   IV access

            i.   hypotensive patient

            ii.   pulmonary edema patient

F.   Documentation

    1.   Documentation of the renal calculi patient

    2.   Documentation of dialysis complication patient

Medicine
Gynecology

AEMT Education Standard

Applies fundamental knowledge to provide basic and selected advanced emergency care and transportation based on assessment findings for an acutely ill patient.

AEMT-Level Instructional Guideline

The AEMT Instructional Guidelines in this section include all the topics and material at the EMT level.

Medicine
Non-Traumatic Musculoskeletal Disorders

AEMT Education Standard

Applies fundamental knowledge to provide basic and selected advanced emergency care and transportation based on assessment findings for an acutely ill patient.

AEMT-Level Instructional Guideline

The AEMT Instructional Guidelines in this section include all the topics and material at the EMT level.

Medicine
Diseases of the Eyes, Ears, Nose, and Throat

AEMT Education Standard

Applies fundamental knowledge to provide basic and selected advanced emergency care and transportation based on assessment findings for an acutely ill patient.

AEMT-Level Instructional Guideline

The AEMT Instructional Guidelines in this section include all the topics and material at the EMT level.

Shock and Resuscitation

AEMT Education Standard

Applies fundamental knowledge to provide basic and selected advanced emergency care and transportation based on assessment findings for a patient in shock, respiratory failure or arrest, cardiac failure or arrest and post resuscitation management.

AEMT-Level Instructional Guideline

The AEMT Instructional Guidelines in this section include all the topics and material at the EMT level PLUS the following material:

I.   Ethical Issues in Resuscitation
      A.   Withholding Resuscitation Attempts
            1.   Irreversible death
            2.   Do Not Resuscitate (DNR) orders
      B.   Provide Emotional Support for Family
      C.   Organ and Tissue Donation

II.   Anatomy and Physiology Review
      A.   Respiratory System
      B.   Cardiovascular System

III.   Cardiac Arrest
      A.   Pathophysiology
            1.   If the heart stops contracting, no blood will flow.
            2.   The body cannot survive when the heart stops.
                  a.   Organ damage begins quickly after the heart stops.
                  b.   Brain damage
                        i.   begins 4-6 minutes after the patient suffers cardiac arrest.
                        ii.   becomes irreversible in 8-10 minutes.
            3.   Cardio-pulmonary resuscitation (CPR)
                  a.   Artificial ventilation
                  b.   External chest compressions
                  c.   Oxygenated blood is circulated to the brain and other vital organs
      B.   General Reasons for the Heart to Stop Beating
            1.   Sudden death and heart disease
            2.   Breathing stops, especially in infants and children
            3.   Medical emergencies
            4.   Trauma

IV.   Resuscitation
   A.   System Components to Maximize Survival
      1.   Early access
         a.   Public education and awareness
            i.   rapid recognition of a cardiac emergency
            ii.   rapid notification before CPR starts - "phone first"
         b.   911-pre-arrival instructions and dispatcher directed CPR
      2.   Early CPR
         a.   Lay public
            i.   family
            ii.   bystanders
         b.   Emergency Medical Responders
      3.   Early Defibrillation
      4.   Early Advanced Care
   B.   Basic Cardiac Life Support (Refer to Current American Heart Association Guidelines)
      1.   Adult CPR and foreign body airway obstruction
      2.   Child CPR and foreign body airway obstruction
      3.   Infant CPR and foreign body airway obstruction
      4.   Neonatal sequence
      5.   Alternative CPR techniques -- Interposed abdominal compression
   C.   Airway Control and Ventilation
      1.   Airway adjuncts
         a.   Basic adjuncts
         b.   Advanced adjuncts (as defined by Scope of Practice)
      2.   Ventilation
         a.   Hazards of over-ventilation
            i.   reduces blood return to the right side of the heart
            ii.   reduces the overall blood flow that can be generated with CPR
         b.   Devices to assist ventilation
   D.   Chest Compressions
      1.   Factors which decrease effectiveness
         a.   Compression that are too shallow
         b.   Slow compression rate
         c.   Sub-maximum recoil
         d.   Frequent interruptions
      2.   Devices to assist circulation
         a.   Active compression-decompression CPR
         b.   Impedance threshold device
         c.   Mechanical piston device
         d.   Load-distributing band or vest CPR

V.   Automated External Defibrillation (AED) -- (Refer To Current American Heart Association Guidelines)
   A.   Adult Sequence

B. Child Sequence
C. Infant Sequence
D. Special Situations
    1. Pacemaker/implanted cardioverter/defibrillator
    2. Wet patients
    3. Transdermal medication patches

VI. Advanced Life Support - Refer to the Current American Heart Association Guidelines

VII. Post-Resuscitation Support - Refer to the Current American Heart Association Guidelines
A. Return of Spontaneous Circulation (ROSC)
    1. Temperature regulation
        a. Induced hypothermia
    2. Glucose control
    3. Organ specific support
        a. Respiratory system
            i. ventilation rates
        b. Cardiovascular system
            i. monitor
            ii. leave AED pads in place
        c. Central nervous system

VIII. Shock
A. Definition
    1. Perfusion is the passage of blood and oxygen and other essential nutrients to the body's cells
    2. While delivering these essentials to the body's cells, the circulatory system is also removing waste such as carbon dioxide from the cells
    3. Shock is a state of hypoperfusion, or inadequate perfusion of blood through body tissues
    4. Hypoperfusion can lead to death if not corrected
B. Anatomy and Physiology Review
    1. Heart/blood vessels
    2. Physiology of respiration
        a. Gas exchange
            i. alveolar level
            ii. tissue level
        b. Circulation
            i. pulmonary
            ii. systemic
    3. Essential components for normal perfusion
        a. Functioning pump/heart
            i. stroke volume
            ii. cardiac output
            iii. blood pressure

                        a)   mean arterial pressure
                        b)   pulse pressure
                iv.   baroreceptors
                v.   nervous control of heart
                        a)   sympathetic nervous system
                        b)   parasympathetic nervous system
        b.   Adequate volume
                i.   formed elements
                ii.   plasma
        c.   Intact container/vessels
                i.   arteries
                ii.   arterioles
                iii.   capillary beds
                iv.   sphincters
                v.   venules
                vi.   veins
                vii.   capacity of each vessel
                viii.   sympathetic nervous system control of each vessel
                ix.   blood flow controlled by cellular tissue demands
                x.   sphincter control
C.   Tissue Hypoperfusion
        1.   Inadequate fluid volume
        2.   Inadequate pump
        3.   Inadequate container size
D.   Physiologic Response to Shock
        1.   Cellular
                a.   Fick principle
                b.   Waste removal
                c.   Aerobic metabolism/glycolosis
                d.   Anaerobic metabolism
        2.   Sympathetic nervous system and endocrine implications
E.   Categories of Shock
        1.   Compensated shock
        2.   Decompensated shock
        3.   Irreversible shock
F.   Specific Types of Shock
        1.   Hypovolemic
                a.   Hemorrhage classifications
                        i.   hemostasis
                        ii.   vascular phase
                        iii.   platelet phase
                        iv.   coagulation phase
                        v.   tension lines
                        vi.   factors affecting clotting/coagulation
                b.   Stages of hemorrhage
                        i.   Class I

     ii. Class II
     iii. Class III
     iv. Class IV
  2. Distributive
    a. Neurogenic
    b. Anaphylactic
    c. Septic
    d. Psychogenic (vasovagal)
  3. Cardiogenic
    a. Intrinsic causes -- heart muscle damage
     i. physiology
     ii. signs/symptoms
     iii. assessment
     iv. management
    b. Extrinsic causes
     i. cardiac tamponade
     ii. tension pneumothorax
  4. Respiratory

G. Complications of Shock
  1. Multiple Organ Dysfunction Syndrome (MODS)
    a. Sepsis
    b. Death of organs
    c. Death of organism
  2. Acute Respiratory Distress Syndrome (ARDS)

H. Patient Assessment
  1. Scene size-up
  2. Perform a primary assessment
  3. Obtains a relevant history
  4. Perform a secondary assessment
  5. Perform a reassessment

I. Management
  1. Manual in-line spinal stabilization, as needed.
  2. Comfort, calm, and reassure the patient
  3. Do not give food or drink
  4. Airway control
  5. Breathing
    a. Assist ventilation, as needed
    b. Oxygen administration (high concentration)
  6. Circulation
    a. Attempt to control obvious external bleeding.
    b. Patient positioning
    c. Keep patient warm - attempt to maintain normal body temperature.
  7. Pneumatic anti-shock garment (PASG) application
  8. Fluid resuscitation
    a. Controllable external hemorrhage
    b. Uncontrollable external hemorrhage
    c. Internal hemorrhage

         9.   Begin transport at the earliest possible moment

        10.   Treat any additional injuries that might be present

J.   Devices to Assist Circulation

IX.   Age-Related Variations

    A.   Pediatrics

       1.   Common causes of shock

          a.   Trauma

          b.   Fluid loss

          c.   Neurological injury

          d.   Anaphylaxis

          e.   Heart disease

          f.   Infection

       2.   Presentation

          a.   Cardiovascular

          b.   Skin signs

          c.   Mental status

          d.   Decreased fluid output

          e.   Vital signs

       3.   Anatomic and physiologic implications

          a.   Unreliable indicators

          b.   Indicators of shock

              i.   tachycardia for age

             ii.   weak distal pulses

             iii.   delayed capillary refill time

             iv.   cool mottled extremities

             v.   altered mental status

       4.   Management

          a.   Inline spinal stabilization

          b.   Suction, as needed

          c.   High-concentration oxygen

          d.   Control bleeding

          e.   Positioning

          f.   Maintain body temperature

          g.   Fluid replacement

          h.   Transport

    B.   Geriatrics

       1.   Assessment

          a.   Body system changes affecting presentation of shock

              i.   nervous system

             ii.   cardiovascular

                  a)   difficulty tolerating hypotension from hemorrhage

                  b)   beta-blocker and calcium channel blockers can alter physiologic response to hemorrhage

             iii.   respiratory

    iv. integumentary

    v. renal

    vi. gastrointestinal

  b. Vital sign variations

    i. altered mental status

      a) sudden onset

      b) other causes

    ii. hypoxia

  c. Airway

    i. decreased cough reflex

    ii. cervical arthritis

    iii. loose dentures

  d. Breathing

    i. higher resting respiratory rate

    ii. lower tidal volume

    iii. less elasticity/compliance of chest wall

  e. Circulation

    i. Higher resting heart rate

    ii. Irregular pulses

  f. Skin

    i. dry, less elastic

    ii. cold

    iii. fever, not common

    iv. hot

2. Management

  a. In-line spinal stabilization

  b. Suction, as needed

  c. High-flow oxygen

  d. Control bleeding

  e. Positioning

  f. Maintain body temperature

3. Transport

Trauma
Trauma Overview

AEMT Education Standard

Applies fundamental knowledge to provide basic and selected advanced emergency care and transportation based on assessment findings for an acutely injured patient.

AEMT-Level Instructional Guideline

The AEMT Instructional Guidelines in this section include all the topics and material at the EMT level.

I. Identification and Categorization of Trauma Patients
    A. Entry-Level Students Need to Be Familiar With:
        1. National Trauma Triage Protocol
            a. Centers for Disease Control and Prevention. Guidelines for Field Triage of Injured Patients: Recommendations of the National Expert Panel on Field Triage. MMWR 2008:58 RR-1:1-35.
            b. http://cdc.gov/fieldtriage contains the National Trauma Triage Protocols and additional instructional materials.

Bleeding

AEMT Education Standard

Applies fundamental knowledge to provide basic and selected advanced emergency care and transportation based on assessment findings for an acutely injured patient.

AEMT-Level Instructional Guideline

The AEMT Instructional Guidelines in this section include all the topics and material at the EMT level.

I.   Fluid Resuscitation in Bleeding and Shock
     A.   Pathophysiology of Shock
          1.   Cardiac control in homeostasis of blood pressure
              a.   Changes in function in hemorrhagic shock
                  i.   rate
                  ii.   volume circulated
                  iii.   preload
                  iv.   afterload
                  v.   Starling's law
                  vi.   cardiac output
              b.   Loss of ability to compensate
          2.   Neurological/Autonomic control in homeostasis
              a.   Vasoconstriction
                  i.   peripheral
                  ii.   central
                  iii.   chemoreceptors
                  iv.   baroreceptors
               b.   Loss of ability to compensate
          3.   Blood vessels in homeostasis of blood
              a.   Neurovascular control
                  i.   chemoreceptors
                  ii.   baroreceptors
               b.   Clotting
              c.   Loss of ability to compensate
     B.   Blood Volume and Shock Stages
          1.   Class I
              a.   Definition
              b.   Estimated blood loss
              c.   Assessment findings
          2.   Class II
              a.   Definition

        b.   Estimated blood loss

        c.   Assessment findings

3.   Class III

        a.   Definition

        b.   Estimated blood loss

        c.   Assessment findings

4.   Class IV

        a.   Definition

        b.   Estimated blood loss

        c.   Assessment findings

C.   Management of Bleeding and Shock Using Fluid Resuscitation

1.   Review of fluid physiology and special considerations in shock

        a.   Oncotic pressure

        b.   Hydrostatic pressure

        c.   Osmosis

        d.   Diffusion

2.   Review of IV skills and special considerations in shock

        a.   Vascular anatomy

        b.   Catheter selection

             i.   diameter impact

             ii.   length impact

        c.   Other considerations

             i.   tubing length and extension tubing

             ii.   impact of saline locks on IV flow

3.   General principles of shock management

        a.   Scene safety

        b.   Body substance isolation

        c.   Rapid transport without unnecessary scene delays

        d.   Airway

        e.   Breathing

             i.   hyperventilation is contraindicated

             ii.   monitor oxygen saturation to maintain above 90%

        f.   Circulation

             i.   control the external bleeding

                 a)   start two large-bore IV's enroute

                 b)   fluid replacement with warmed isotonic solution up to 30 ml/kg in 250 - 500 ml increments with frequent reassessments

                 c)   monitor response to therapy

             ii.   internal bleeding and non-compressible bleeding

                 a)   position the patient to maximize perfusion

                 b)   consider PASG by protocol

                 c)   start two large-bore IV's enroute

                 d)   fluid replacement with warmed isotonic solution up to 20-30 ml/kg in boluses of 250-500 ml

                 e)   maintain blood pressure between 70mm/hg and 90 mm/hg

4. Reassessment of fluid therapy after initial treatment
    a. Rapid return to normal vitals and vitals remain normal
        i. slow IV to TKO rate
        ii. reassess often
    b. Inconsistent response to initial treatment with initial improvement followed by slow deterioration
        i. indicates ongoing uncontrolled blood loss
        ii. maintain blood pressure between 70-90mm/Hg depending on local protocol

II. Special Considerations in Fluid Resuscitation
  A. Permissive Hypotension
  B. Reperfusion Injury
  C. Pediatrics
    1. Temperature control is critical in maintaining perfusion
    2. Use of IV is for known required fluid replacement
    3. Consider use of IO if peripheral vein is not accessible and patient is in immediate need of fluid
        a. Keep normal vital signs by age on hand
        b. Infuse up to 20cc/kg of warmed isotonic solution
        c. Consider a second infusion of 20cc/kg if there is no response to first
        d. Second infusion should be done keeping in mind that the patient needs rapid restoration of red blood cells while awaiting definitive care if shock is due to non-compressible hemorrhage
        e. A third infusion of 20cc/kg may be considered in patients with controlled hemorrhage
        f. The use of continuous infusion in uncontrolled hemorrhage should be done to maintain adequate perfusion levels of critical organs enroute to the hospital
  D. Geriatrics
    1. Patients with chronic hypertension may have higher blood pressure value needs to achieve the same level of end organ perfusion than other patients
        a. Patient may be in shock with blood pressure above 100
        b. Modest amounts of blood loss can lead to shock
            i. reduced blood volume
            ii. possible anemia
        c. Patient is less able to tolerate excessive fluids
            i. possible anemia
            ii. possible electrolyte alterations
  E. Obstetrical Patients
    1. Shock states lead to shunting of blood away from fetus
    2. The closer the maternal blood pressure is to normal, the better the fetal perfusion

Trauma
Chest Trauma

AEMT Education Standard

Applies fundamental knowledge to provide basic and selected advanced emergency care and transportation based on assessment findings for an acutely injured patient.

AEMT-Level Instructional Guideline

The AEMT Instructional Guidelines in this section include all the topics and material at the EMT level PLUS the following material:

I.   Traumatic Aortic Disruption
        A.   Pathophysiology
                1.   Role of deceleration and speed as MOI
                2.   Partial tear
                3.   Complete tear
        B.   Assessment
                1.   Mechanism of injury
                2.   High percent have no signs of external chest trauma
                3.   Hypotension
                4.   Signs of Shock
                5.   Chest pain – tearing in nature
                6.   Suspicion raises with chest wall injury
                7.   Unusual pulses or blood pressure in upper extremities
                8.   Voice changes
                        a.   Hoarseness
                        b.   Stridor
                9.   Difficulty swallowing
        C.   Management
                1.   Review knowledge from previous levels
                2.   AVO management
                3.   High index of suspicion based upon MOI
                4.   Do not over-hydrate

II.   Pulmonary Contusion
        A.   Pathophysiology
                1.   Blunt trauma with associated injuries (rib fractures)
                2.   Capillary leakage into alveoli prevents gas exchange
                3.   Decrease lung compliance
                4.   Slowly developing process
                5.   Diffuse vs localized

B.   Assessment
1. Respiratory distress symptoms
2. Hemoptysis
3. Chest pain from blunt trauma
4. Cough
5. rales or rhonchi
6. Hypoxia
7. High index of suspicion based on MOI
C.   Management
1. AVO management
2. IV fluid administration – over hydration is contraindicated (see Trauma: Bleeding

III.   Blunt Cardiac Injury
A.   Pathophysiology
1. Cardiac arrhythmias sometimes occur
2. Heart failure may occur
    a. Review of right sided heart failure
    b. Review of left-sided heart failure
B.   Assessment
1. High index of suspicion with anterior blunt chest trauma
2. Clinical signs vary due to injury location in heart – vessels, muscle mass or conduction system
3. Tachycardia
4. May not exhibit external chest discoloration
5. Chest pain – retrosternal (MI type pain)
C.   Management
1. High index of suspicion
2. AVO management
3. Limit fluids if signs of heart failure are present
    a. lung crackles
    b. Jugular venous distension
4. Be prepared for deteriorations in patients with rapid or irregular pulses

IV.   Hemothorax
A.   Pathophysiology
1. Review knowledge from previous levels
2. Penetrating wounds
    a. Tears in lung parenchyma
    b. Puncture great vessels or heart
3. Clotting in the chest may release fibrolysins – continue bleeding process
4. Loss of circulating blood in vessels
B.   Assessment
1. Review knowledge from previous levels
2. Shock
3. Unequal breath sounds

4. Dullness on percussion
5. Jugular venous distention assessment
 a. Proper patient positioning for jugular venous assessment
 b. Flat with hypovolemia
 c. Distended if increased intrathoracic pressure

C. Management
 1. Review knowledge from previous levels
 2. AVO management
 3. Fluid bolus and continued hypovolemia assessment (see Trauma: Bleeding
 4. Rapid transport to appropriate facility

V. Pneumothorax
 A. Open
  1. Pathophysiology
   a. Review knowledge from previous levels
   b. Open wound to the chest wall
   c. Fracture of chest wall structure
   d. Hypoxia
   e. Loss of lung adhesion to chest wall due to loss of surface tension-collapse of lung
  2. Assessment
   a. Review knowledge from previous levels
   b. AVO assessment
   c. Chest Assessment
    i. inspection
    ii. auscultation
    iii. percussion
   d. Subcutaneous emphysema
   e. Hypovolemia signs
   f. Cardiac dysrhythmia
  3. Management
   a. Review knowledge from previous levels
   b. Airway, respiration and ventilation management
   c. Inspect chest
    i. cover open wounds with non-porous dressing
    ii. excessive pressure ventilation can cause tension pneumothorax
   d. Pneumothorax complications
   e. Dysrhythmia treatment
 B. Simple
  1. Pathophysiology
   a. Review knowledge from previous levels
   b. Defect in chest wall allow air to enter pleural space
   c. Some low velocity wounds self-seal

    d. If chest wall hole is 2/3 size of trachea, more air will enter from the atmosphere – sucking sound will be present

    e. With large holes air enters both the trachea and the hole rapidly collapsing the lung

    f. Delayed or improper treatment will lead to tension pneumothorax with large open wounds

  2. Assessment

    a. Review knowledge from previous levels

    b. AVO assessment

    c. Chest Assessment

      i. inspection

        a) immediately cover open wounds with nonporous dressings

      ii. auscultation

        a) unequal breath sounds

      iii. percussion

    d. Subcutaneous emphysema

    e. Hypovolemia signs

    f. Cardiac dysrhythmia

  3. Management

    a. Review knowledge from previous levels

    b. Airway, respiration and ventilation management

    c. Inspect chest

      i. cover open wounds with non-porous dressing

      ii. excessive pressure ventilation can cause tension pneumothorax

    d. Pneumothorax complications

    e. Dysrhythmia treatment

C. Tension

  1. Pathophysiology

    a. Review knowledge of previous levels

    b. Formation of one-way valve – air from either lungs or atmosphere

    c. Increased pleural pressure – shift of mediastinal structures to contralateral side – causes kinking of great veins decreasing cardiac output

    d. May be closed – untreated rupture of alveolar sac

    e. May be open – penetrating trauma – injury to bronchus or bronchi

  2. Assessment

    a. Review knowledge of previous levels

    b. Severe respiratory distress

    c. Jugular vein distention

    d. Deviation of the trachea

      i. almost never seen in the prehospital environment

      ii. more easily seen on x-ray.

    e. Tachycardia

    f. Narrow pulse pressure

        g.   Absent breath sounds on affected side

        h.   Unequal chest rise

3.   Management

    a.   Review knowledge from previous levels

    b.   Airway, respiration and ventilation management

    c.   Inspect chest

        i.   cover open wounds with non-porous dressing

        ii.   excessive pressure ventilation can cause tension pneumothorax

    d.   Pneumothorax complications

    e.   Dysrhythmia treatment

VI.   Cardiac Tamponade

    A.   Pathophysiology

        1.   Review knowledge from previous levels

        2.   Mechanism of injury

            a.   Penetrating trauma

            b.   Much more rare in blunt trauma

        3.   Blood in the pericardial sac

            a.   Perforation of heart muscle

            b.   Amount of blood dependent in where blood originates

            c.   Sac is not elastic – no stretching

            d.   Small amounts (55cc) can cause reduction in cardiac output

            e.   Increased sac pressure puts pressure on coronary arteries

    B.   Assessment

        1.   Jugular vein distention – increase in CVP

        2.   Increased diastolic pressure

        3.   Narrowed pulse pressure

    C.   Management

    a.   Review knowledge from previous levels

    b.   Airway, respiration and ventilation management

    c.   Inspect chest

        i.   cover open wounds with non-porous dressing

        ii.   excessive pressure ventilation can cause tension pneumothorax

    d.   Rapid IV fluid bolus

    e.   Dysrhythmia treatment

VII.   Rib Fractures

    A.   Pathophysiology

    B.   Assessment

    C.   Management

VIII. Flail Chest
      A. Pathophysiology
      B. Assessment
      C. Management

IX. Commotio Cordis
      A. Pathophysiology
      B. Assessment
      C. Management

Trauma
Abdominal and Genitourinary Trauma

AEMT Education Standard

Applies fundamental knowledge to provide basic and selected advanced emergency care and transportation based on assessment findings for an acutely injured patient.

AEMT-Level Instructional Guideline

The AEMT Instructional Guidelines in this section include all the topics and material at the EMT level PLUS the following material:

I.   Incidence
    A.   Morbidity/Mortality

II.   Anatomy
    A.   Quadrants and Boundaries of the Abdomen
    B.   Surface Anatomy of the Abdomen
    C.   Intraperitoneal Structures
    D.   Retroperitoneal Structures
    E.   Reproductive Organs

III. Physiology
    A.   Solid Organs
    B.   Hollow Organs
    C.   Vascular Structures

IV.   Specific Injuries
    A.   Closed Abdominal Trauma
        1.   Mechanism of injury
            a.   Compression
            b.   Deceleration
            c.   MVA
            d.   Motorcycle collisions
            e.   Pedestrian injuries
            f.   Falls
            g.   Assault
            h.   Blast injuries
        2.   Signs and Symptoms
            a.   Pain
            b.   Guarding
            c.   Distention – rise in abdomen between pubis and xiphoid process
            d.   Discoloration of abdominal wall

        e.   Tenderness – on movement

        f.   Lower rib fractures

        g.   May be overlooked in multi-system injuries

        h.   Suspicion based on mechanism of injury

3.   Assessment

        a.   Inspection

        b.   Noting position of the patient

        c.   Noting pain with movement

        d.   Auscultation – little value

        e.   Blood loss through rectum or vomit

4.   Management

        a.   Oxygen

        b.   Transport in position of comfort if indicated

        c.   Treat for shock – internal bleeding

B.   Penetrating/Open Abdominal Trauma

1.   Low velocity penetration – knife wound, tear of abdominal wall, consider injury to underlying organ

2.   Medium velocity penetration – shot gun wound

3.   High-velocity penetration – gunshot wound

4.   Signs and Symptoms of penetrating abdominal trauma

        a.   Bleeding

        b.   Puncture wounds – entrance and exits

        c.   Many signs and symptoms of closed abdominal wounds could also be present along with a puncture wound

5.   Assessment

        a.   Clothing removal

        b.   Inspection – look for exit wounds including posterior

        c.   Noting position of patient

6.   Management

        a.   Cover wounds

        b.   Use non-porous dressing if chest may be involved

        c.   Treat for shock

        d.   Oxygen

        e.   Transport decision

C.   Considerations in Abdominal Trauma

1.   Hollow organs injuries

        a.   Stomach

        b.   Small bowel

        c.   Large bowel

        d.   Gallbladders

        e.   Urinary bladder

        f.   Considerations of signs and symptoms of hollow organ injuries

                i.   pain – may be intense with open wounds to the stomach or small bowel

                ii.   infection – delayed complication which may be fatal

                iii.   air in peritoneal cavity

2. Solid organ injuries
    a. Blood in the abdomen does not acutely produce abdominal pain
    b. Abdominal pain from solid organ penetration or rupture is of slow onset
    c. Liver
        i. largest organ
        ii. very vascular leading to hypo-perfusion
        iii. injured with lower right rib fractures or penetrating trauma
    d. Spleen
        i. injured in auto crashes, falls, bicycle accidents, motorcycles
        ii. injured with lower left rib fractures or penetrating trauma
        iii. left shoulder pain
    e. Pancreas
    f. Kidney
        i. vascular
        ii. blood in urine
    g. Diaphragm
        i. abnormal respiratory sounds
        ii. shortness of breath
    h. Retroperitoneal structures

V. General Assessment
    A. High Index of Suspicion
    B. Pain With Abdominal Trauma Is Often Masked Due to Other Injuries
    C. Airway Patency
    D. External and Internal Hemorrhage
    E. Identification and Management of Life Threats
    F. Spinal Immobilization
    G. Physical Exam
        1. Inspection
        2. Auscultation
        3. Palpation
    H. Associated Trauma
    I. Recognition and Prevention of Shock
    J. PASG for Pelvic Fracture Stabilization
    K. Transportation Decisions to Appropriate Facility

VI. General Management
    A. Scene Safety/Standard Precautions
    B. Airway Management
    C. Oxygenation and Ventilation
    D. Spinal Immobilization Considerations
    E. Control External Hemorrhage
    F. Identification of Life Threatening Injury
    G. Application and Inflation of PASG for Pelvic Fracture Stabilization
    H. Abdominal Trauma May Be Masked by Other Body System Trauma

I. Transportation to Appropriate Facility
   1. No transport decisions
   2. Transport to acute care facility
   3. Transport to trauma center
   4. ALS mutual aid
J. Communication and Documentation

VII. Age-Related Variations for Pediatric and Geriatric Assessment and Management
   A. Pediatric
      1. Mechanism of injury as pedestrian
      2. Use of PASG (fracture stabilization)
   B. Geriatric

VIII. Special Considerations of Abdominal Trauma
   A. Sexual Assault
      1. Criminal implications and evidence management
      2. Patient confidentiality
      3. Treat wounds as other soft tissue injuries
   B. Vaginal Bleeding Due to Trauma
      1. May be due to penetrating or blunt trauma
      2. Assess to determine pregnancy
      3. Apply sterile absorbent vaginal pad
      4. Determine mechanism of injury
      5. Do not insert gloved fingers for instruments in vagina

Trauma
Orthopedic Trauma

AEMT Education Standard

Applies fundamental knowledge to provide basic and selected advanced emergency care and transportation based on assessment findings for an acutely injured patient.

AEMT-Level Instructional Guideline

The AEMT Instructional Guidelines in this section include all the topics and material at the EMT level PLUS the following material:

I.   Amputations
    A.   Pathophysiology
        1.   Tear, retraction and spasm of blood vessels
        2.   Amputated extremity
        3.   Re-implantation opportunities
    B.   Special Assessment Finding
        1.   Location of amputation
        2.   Tearing versus cutting amputations
        3.   Assessment of amputated part
    C.   Special Management Considerations
        1.   Tourniquet
        2.   Fluid replacement

II.   Pelvic Fractures
    A.   Anatomy of the Pelvic Girdle
    B.   Pathophysiology
        1.   Type I fractures
            a.   avulsion fractures
            b.   fracture of pubis or ischium
            c.   fracture of iliac wing
            d.   fracture of sacrum
            e.   fracture of coccyx
        2.   Type II fractures
            a.   Single fracture of pelvic ring
            b.   unilateral fractures of both pelvic rami
            c.   Subluxation of the symphysis pubis
            d.   Fracture near the sacroiliac joint
        3.   Type III fractures
        4.   Type IV fractures

5.   Associated injuries
      a.   potential blood loss amounts
      b.   retroperitoneal space potential blood loss amounts
6.   Significance of posterior fractures

C.   Special Assessment Findings
1.   Pelvic instability
2.   Pain
3.   Rectal bleeding

D.   Management Considerations
1.   Stabilize with PASG and longboard to minimize movement
2.   Specialized pelvic immobilization devices
3.   Management of blood loss

III.   Compartment Syndrome

A.   Pathophysiology
1.   Review previous knowledge
2.   Locally increased pressure compromises local circulation and neuromuscular function
3.   Occur with crush injuries
4.   Burns
5.   Tight casts as part of fracture management
6.   Occlusion of arterial blood supply
7.   Snake bites
8.   Rhabdomyolysis

B.   Special Assessment Findings
1.   Review previous knowledge
2.   Severe limb pain
3.   Muscle compartment extremely tight
4.   Decreased sensation to touch
5.   Paresthesia
6.   Loss of distal circulation
7.   Paralysis

C.   Special Management Considerations
1.   Review previous knowledge
2.   Removal of plaster casts
3.   Elevation
4.   Ice
5.   Rapid transport to appropriate facility
6.   Treatment of acidemia
7.   Treatment of Rhabdomyolysis
8.   Pain Management

Trauma
Soft Tissue Trauma

AEMT Education Standard

Applies fundamental knowledge to provide basic and selected advanced emergency care and transportation based on assessment findings for an acutely injured patient.

AEMT-Level Instructional Guideline

The AEMT Instructional Guidelines in this section include all the topics and material at the EMT level PLUS the following material:

I. Incidence of Soft Tissue Injury
    A. Mortality/Morbidity

II. Anatomy and Physiology of Soft Tissue Injury
    A. Layers of the Skin
    B. Function of the Skin

III. Closed Soft Tissue Injury
    A. Type of Injuries
        1. Contusion
        2. Hematoma
        3. Crush injuries
    B. Signs and Symptoms
        1. Discoloration
        2. Swelling
        3. Pain
    C. Assessment
        1. Mechanism of injury, suspect underlying organ trauma/injury
        2. Diffuse or generalized soft tissue trauma can be critical
        3. Pulse, movement, sensation
    D. Management
        1. Ice
        2. Splinting if necessary

IV. Open Soft Tissue Injury
    A. Type of Injuries
        1. Abrasions
        2. Lacerations
        3. Avulsions
        4. Bites
        5. Impaled objects

          6.   Amputations

          7.   Blast injuries/High Pressure

          8.   Penetrating/Punctures

B.   Complications of Soft Tissue Injury

          1.   Blood loss – review bleeding and shock

          2.   Infection

                a.   Mechanisms of infection

                b.   Risk factors

C.   Signs and Symptoms of Open Soft Tissue Injuries

          1.   Bleeding and Shock, Chest Trauma and other sections in trauma discuss many of the signs and symptoms of injuries to those areas that also include a soft tissue injury

          2.   Pain

          3.   Hemorrhage

          4.   Contaminated wounds

          5.   Impaled objects

          6.   Loss of extremity

          7.   Entrance and exit wounds

          8.   Flap of skin attached

V.   General Assessment

      A.   Safety of Environment/Standard Precautions

      B.   Airway Patency

      C.   Respiratory Distress

      D.   Concepts of Open Wound Dressings/Bandaging

          1.   Sterile

          2.   Non-sterile

          3.   Occlusive

          4.   Non-occlusive

          5.   Wet

          6.   Dry

          7.   Tourniquet

          8.   Complications of dressings/bandages

      E.   Hemorrhage Control

          1.   Severity of injury

          2.   Elevation

          3.   Pressure dressing

          4.   Pressure points

          5.   Tourniquets

      F.   Associated Injuries

          1.   Airway

          2.   Face

          3.   Neck

VI.   Management
    A.   Airway Management
    B.   Control Hemorrhage
    C.   Prevention of Shock
    D.   Prevent Infection
    E.   Transportation to the Appropriate Facility
    F.   Communication and Documentation
    G.   Bites
        1.   Control hemorrhage
        2.   Cat and human bites often lead to serious infection
    H.   Avulsions
        1.   Never remove skin flap regardless of size
        2.   Complete avulsion often has serious infection concerns
        3.   Place skin in anatomic position if flat avulsion

VII.   Incidence of Burn Injury
    A.   Morbidity/Mortality
    B.   Risk Factors

VIII. Anatomy and Physiology of Burns
    A.   Types of Burns
        1.   Thermal
        2.   Inhalation
        3.   Chemical
        4.   Electrical
    B.   Complications of Burns
        1.   Thermal
            a.   Exposure time
            b.   Enclosed space vs open
            c.   Scalds with unusual history patterns may be abuse
        2.   Inhalation
            a.   Airway closure due to swelling may be very rapid
            b.   Carbon monoxide inhalation
        3.   Chemical
            a.   Acid and alkaline are different
            b.   Solutions and powders are different
        4.   Electrical
            a.   Skin inspection may be not indicate seriousness of burn
            b.   Entrance and exit wounds
            c.   Current across chest may cause cardiac arrest
            d.   Lighting strikes may cause cardiac arrest
    C.   Depth Classification of Burns
        1.   Superficial
        2.   Partial-thickness
        3.   Full-thickness

D. Body Surface Area of Burns
   1. 'rule of nines'
   2. 'rule of ones'
E. Severity of Burns
   1. Minor
   2. Moderate
   3. Severe

IX. Complications of Burn Injuries
   A. Infection
   B. Vasoconstriction
   C. Hypoxia
   D. Hypothermia
   E. Hypovolemia
   F. Complications With Circumferential Burns
   G. Pediatric/Geriatric Abuse

X. General Assessment of Burn Injuries
   A. Safety/Standard Precautions
   B. Airway Patency
   C. Respiratory Distress
   D. Hemorrhage Control
   E. Classification of Burn Depth
   F. Percentage of Body Surface Area Affected
   G. Severity

XI. General Management
   A. Stop the Burning
   B. Airway Management
   C. Respiratory Distress
   D. Circulatory
   E. Dry, Sterile, Non-Adherent Dressing
   F. Remove Jewelry and Clothing
   G. Prevent Shock
   H. Prevent Hypothermia
   I. Transportation to Appropriate Facility
      1. ALS mutual aid
      2. Criteria for burn unit
   J. Pediatric Considerations
   K. Geriatric Considerations

XII. Specific Burn Injury Management Considerations
   A. Thermal
      1. Complete general management
      2. May be associated with an inhalation injury
      3. Large BSB also have hypovolemia and hypothermia

4. Cool small or those remaining hot
5. Dry dressing help prevent infection and provide comfort
6. Time in contact with heat increases damage
- B. Inhalation
    1. Complications are related to chemicals within inhaled air
    2. Edema of mucosa of airway can be rapid – need ALS backup if signs and symptoms of edema are present, such as voice change, singed nasal hairs, etc
    3. Percent of oxygen in ambient air is different so hypoxia, and carbon monoxide or other chemicals may enter the blood
    4. Burns in enclosed spaces without ventilation cause inhalation injuries
- C. Chemical
    1. Some burns are liquid and need copious amounts of flushing with water
    2. Some burns are powders and need brushed off to remove chemicals
    3. Chemical burns treatments can be specific to the burning agent and labels should be read
    4. Burns at industrial sites may have experts available on scene
- D. Electrical
    1. The type of electric current, amperage and volts, have effect on seriousness of burns
    2. No patient should be touched while in contact with current
    3. Sometimes electric current crosses the chest and causes cardiac arrest or arrhythmias
    4. Many underlying injuries to organs and the nervous system may be present
    5. Radiation burns require special rescue techniques

XIII. Age-Related Variations
- A. Pediatric
    1. Percentage of surface area in a burn patient
    2. Alteration in calculating the burned area
- B. Geriatrics

Trauma
Head, Facial, Neck, and Spine Trauma

Applies fundamental knowledge to provide basic and selected advanced emergency care and transportation based on assessment findings for an acutely injured patient.

AEMT-Level Instructional Guideline

The AEMT Instructional Guidelines in this section include all the topics and material at the EMT level PLUS the following material:

I. Facial Fractures
    A. Types
        1. Soft tissue injuries
        2. Fractures of facial bones
        3. Eye injuries
        4. Oral/dental injuries
            a. Mandibular fractures
            b. Maxillar fractures
    B. Unstable Facial Fractures
        1. Pathophysiology
            a. Categories of unstable facial fractures
                i. Le Fort I - Fracture separates hard palate and lower maxilla from remainder of skill
                ii. Le Fort II - Fracture separates the nasal and lower maxilla from the facial skull and remainder of the cranial bones
                iii. Le Fort III (craniofacial disjunction) - Fracture separates the entire midface from the cranium.
            b. Blunt trauma to the facial area most frequent cause
        2. Specific assessment considerations
            a. Facial instability
            b. Epistaxis
            c. Edema
            d. Pain
        3. Specific management considerations
            a. Simple airway maneuvers are difficult
            b. Intubation is method of choice for airway protection
            c. Ventilation without intubation is difficult
            d. Manual in-line intubation
            e. Bleeding into the oral cavity; suction
            f. Cricothyroidotomy if indicated
            g. Soft tissue bleeding

C. Signs/Symptoms
    1. Soft tissue injuries are similar to others, but swelling may be more severe.
    2. Facial bones may fracture causing airway and ventilation complications
    3. Eye injuries suffer soft tissue type injuries, abrasions, lacerations, punctures, chemical burns, etc
    4. Eye injuries may cause vision disturbances
    5. Eyes injured with chemicals need flushing with copious amounts of water
    6. Excessive pressure on the eye may "blow out" bones in the orbit
    7. Nasal fractures may cause bleeding
    8. Oral injuries may cause airway management complications

D. Assessment Considerations in Facial and Eye Injuries
    1. Inspection
        a. Open wounds
        b. Swelling
        c. Deformity of bones
        d. Eye clarity without foreign objects
        e. Eye symmetry
        f. Bone alignment in anatomical position
    2. Palpation
    3. Eye examination
        a. Follows finger up, down, lateral
        b. Can read regular print
        c. No blood visible in iris area

E. Management Considerations in Facial and Eye Injuries
    1. Airway must remain open throughout care
    2. Nasopharyngeal airways are contraindicated
    3. Suctioning may be frequent
    4. Broken teeth need to be brought to hospital with patient
    5. Eyes with chemical burns may need to be flushed with copious amounts of water
    6. Simple nose bleeds can be controlled by pinching nostrils
    7. Eye injuries require patching of both eyes
    8. Impaled objects in the eye must be stabilized
    9. Impaled objects in cheeks may be removed
    10. Patients with these injuries may be more comfortable sitting up
    11. Bandaging should not occlude the mouth

II. Laryngeotracheal Injuries
A. Pathophysiology
    1. Trauma directly to structures
    2. Edema
    3. Hemorrhage
B. Specific Assessment Considerations
    1. Swelling
    2. Voice changes
    3. Hemoptyosis

4. Subcutaneous emphysema
5. Structural irregularity
C. Specific Management Considerations
   1. AVO
      a. Airway obstruction common
      b. Careful two man ventilation with bag/valve/mask
         i. may multiple people to maintain effective seal
         ii. may need frequent suctioning
         iii. may need immediate surgical intervention at hospital do not delay transport
      c. Consider advanced airway in apnea
   2. Combative patients
         i. increased intracranial pressure
         ii. hypoxia

III. Laryngeotracheal Injuries
  A. Pathophysiology
   1. Trauma directly to structures
   2. Edema
   3. Hemorrhage
  B. Specific Assessment Considerations
   1. Swelling
   2. Voice changes
   3. hemoptyosis
   4. subcutaneous emphysema
   5. structural irregularity
  C. Specific Management Considerations
   1. AVO
      a. Airway obstruction common
      b. May need surgical airway
   2. Supportive multi-system care

Trauma
Nervous System Trauma

Applies fundamental knowledge to provide basic and selected advanced emergency care and transportation based on assessment findings for an acutely injured patient.

AEMT-Level Instructional Guideline

The AEMT Instructional Guidelines in this section include all the topics and material at the EMT level PLUS the following material:

I.   Incidence of Traumatic Brain Injury
        A.   Morbidity/Mortality
        B.   Prevention Strategies

II.   Traumatic Brain Injury
        A.   Anatomy
                1.   Review of major structures of the brain
                2.   Review of circulation in the brain
        B.   Physiology
                1.   Review of function of brain
        C.   Pathophysiology
                1.   Normal oxygen demand of brain
                        a.   Limited oxygen storing capacity
                        b.   Consequences of oxygen loss
                2.   Role of gas concentrations in vascular diameter
                        a.   Carbon dioxide and vasodilation
                        b.   Oxygen and vasoconstriction
                3.   Brain injury categories
                        a.   Primary brain injury
                        b.   Secondary brain injury
                        c.   Coup/contracoup pattern
                4.   Increasing intracranial pressure
                        a.   Definition
                        b.   Effects
                        c.   Role of mean arterial pressure in maintaining perfusion
                5.   Coma
                        a.   Definition
                        b.   Posturing (decerebrate, decorticate)
                        c.   Normal intracranial pressure (2 – 12 mmHg)

6. Brain herniation
    a. Definition
    b. Effects (i.e. Cushing's triad)
7. Types of brain injuries
    a. Concussion
    b. Diffuse axonal injury
    c. Contusion
    d. Subdural hematoma
    e. Epidural hematoma
    f. Subarachnoid hemorrhage
    g. Intracerebral hemorrhage
    h. Penetrating brain trauma
8. Associated Injuries -- Skull fractures
    a. Linear
    b. Depressed
    c. Open
    d. Basilar

D. Specific Assessment Considerations
1. Level of Consciousness
    a. Signs of increasing intracranial pressure
    b. Cerebral function
    c. Cerebellar function
    d. Cranial nerve function
        i. pupil changes
        ii. doll's eyes
    e. Peripheral/Motor function
2. AVO
    a. Alterations to respiratory and ventilatory effort
    b. Spinal Concerns
3. Vital sign irregularities
    a. Blood pressure changes in intracranial pressure
        i. early
        ii. late
4. Posturing
    a. Types
    b. Significance
5. CSF presence
    a. Causes
    b. Significance
6. Coma assessment
    a. Glasgow Coma Scale
    b. Neurological exam
        i. pupils
        ii. reflexes

E.   Special Management Considerations
        1.   AVO with spinal precautions/immobilization
        2.   Ventilate/assist to maintain PaO2 of 90mmHg
                a.   Cheyne-Strokes respirations
                b.   Irregular or slow respirations
        3.   Seizure precautions
        4.   Fluid management
                a.   Isolated head trauma
                b.   Multisystem trauma with hypovolemia
                c.   role of fluids in managing ICP
        5.   Role of hypothermia in coma

Trauma
Special Considerations in Trauma

AEMT Education Standard

Applies fundamental knowledge to provide basic and selected advanced emergency care and transportation based on assessment findings for an acutely injured patient.

AEMT-Level Instructional Guideline

The AEMT Instructional Guidelines in this section include all the topics and material at the EMT level PLUS the following material:

I.   Trauma in Pregnancy
    A.   Incidence
        1.   Mortality/morbidity
        2.   Risk factors
        3.   Prevention
    B.   Anatomy
        1.   Review of anatomical changes in pregnancy
            a.   Organ displacement
            b.   Organs of pregnancy
            c.   Stages of fetal development/size
    C.   Physiology
        1.   Review of physiological changes in pregnancy
            a.   Respiratory
            b.   cardiovascular
    D.   Pathophysiology
        1.   Shock in pregnancy
            a.   Effects on mother
                i.   shunting
                ii.   increased volume requirements
                iii.   changes in usual findings
            b.   Effects on fetus
        2.   Traumatic abruptio placenta
            a.   Mechanisms of injury
            b.   Effects on mother
            c.   Effects on fetus
        3.   Abdominal injuries
            a.   Mechanisms of injury
            b.   Effects on mother
            c.   Effects on fetus
        4.   Pelvic fracture
            a.   Mechanisms of injury

           b.   Effects on mother

           c.   Effects on fetus

     5.   Seat belt injuries

           a.   Mechanisms of injury

           b.   Effects on mother

           c.   Effects on fetus

     6.   Sexual assault

           a.   Mechanisms of injury

           b.   Effects on mother

           c.   Effects on fetus

E.   Special Considerations in Assessment

     1.   Increased heart rate is not an early sign of hypovolemic shock

     2.   Significant blood loss may not be reflective of usual signs of shock

     3.   Respiratory rate less than 20 should not be considered adequate ventilation

     4.   Loss of landmarks for chest compressions in arrest

     5.   Signs of abruption placentae

     6.   Estimating gestational age of fetus

           a.   Palpation of uterine fundus

           b.   Auscultaton of fetal heart tones

                i.   stethoscope position

                ii.   uterine pulse

F.   Special Considerations in Management

     1.   AVO

           a.   Restriction of diaphragm in mother

                i.   fetal size

                ii.   maternal position

     2.   Circulation

           a.   Fetal pressure on great vessels

                i.   impact on spinal precautions

                ii.   impact on fluid replacement requirements

           b.   IV and fluid management

                i.   the closer the maternal blood pressure is to normal, the better the fetal perfusion

                ii.   normal blood pressure varies by trimester

     3.   Traumatic arrest

           a.   Treatment decisions

           b.   Transport decisions

           c.   Alterations to CPR

                i.   increased airway pressures

                ii.   decreased diaphragm excursion

                iii.   effects on airway management

                      a)   BVM management

                      b)   advanced airway management

II.   Pediatric Trauma
    A.   Incidence
        1.   Mortality/morbidity
            a.   Accidental
            b.   Intentional
        2.   Risk factors
        3.   Prevention
    B.   Anatomy
        1.   Review of anatomical differences by age
            a.   Newborn
            b.   Infant
            c.   Child
                 i.   preschool
                ii.   school-age
                iii.   adolescent
        2.   Review of impact of differences on care
    C.   Physiology
        1.   Review of anatomical differences by age
            a.   Cardiac differences
            b.   Catecholamine regulation
            c.   Review of impact of differences on care
    D.   Pathophysiology
        1.   Alterations to response of shock in the child
        2.   Alterations to response of head injury in the newborn/child
        3.   Alterations to response of spine to injury in the child (i.e. Spinal Cord Injury Without Radiographic Abnormality)
        4.   Alterations to response to chest injury in the child
            a.   Very compliant
            b.   Injury requires great force
            c.   Sudden impact of blunt force to the chest resulting in cardiac dysfunction, even death
            d.   Alterations to response to abdominal injuries in the child
            e.   Relatively larger solid organs
            f.   Less protection from ribs
            g.   Weaker abdominal muscles
        5.   Musculoskeletal
            a.   Damage to epiphyseal plate
            b.   Damage to bone matrix
    E.   Special Considerations in Assessment
        1.   Airway, Breathing, and Circulation
            a.   Review of pediatric anatomy
            b.   Review of normal ventilatory effort in the child
            c.   Review of signs of respiratory distress in child
        2.   Circulation
            a.   Hypotension appears late, use other signs of inadequate circulation
            b.   Capillary refill may be helpful

          c.   Inadequate oxygenation cause bradycardia

          d.   Level of Consciousness may indicate inadequate circulation

                i.   BP estimated as 80 + 2 times the age

                ii.   80ml/Kg blood loss can cause shock

3.   Neurological

          a.   Glasgow Coma Score less than 8 means increased ICP

          b.   Beware of shaken baby syndrome

4.   Head

          a.   Very vascular, even scalp laceration can cause shock

          b.   Falls less than 5 feet are significant

5.   Chest

          a.   Significant internal injury can be present without any external signs

          b.   Tension-pneumothorax is difficult to evaluate

6.   Abdomen

          a.   Spleen most common injured

          b.   Cullen's sign

          c.   Kehr's sign

F.   Special Considerations in Management

1.   Airway, Breathing, and Circulation (improper management is the most common cause of preventable pediatric death)

          a.   High-concentration oxygen and saturation

          b.   Proper advanced airway tube selection

2.   Circulation

          a.   IV selection in the pediatric trauma selection

                i.   site selection

                ii.   access type

                    a)   peripheral

                iii.   keep normal vital signs by age on hand

                iv.   infuse up to 20cc/kg of warmed isotonic solution

                v.   consider a second infusion of 20cc/kg if there is no response to first

                vi.   second infusion should be done keeping in mind that the patient needs rapid restoration of red blood cells while awaiting definitive care if shock is due to non-compressible hemorrhage

                vii.   third infusion of 20cc/kg may be considered in patients with controlled hemorrhage

                viii.   use of continuous infusion in uncontrolled hemorrhage should be done to maintain adequate perfusion levels of critical organs enroute to the hospital

                ix.   maintain body heat to prevent more rapid deterioration

          b.   Fluid replacement

III.	Geriatric Trauma
    A.	Incidence
        1.	Mortality/morbidity
            a.	Accidental
            b.	Intentional
        2.	Risk factors
        3.	Prevention
    B.	Review of Anatomical Changes of Aging
    C.	Review of Physiological Changes of Aging Affecting Trauma
        1.	Respiratory
            a.	Chest wall less compliant
            b.	Less vital capacity
            c.	Decrease in ciliary action
        2.	Cardiovascular
            a.	Heart rate and stroke volume decrease
            b.	Dysrthythmia changes
        3.	Neurological system
            a.	Neuron mass reduction
            b.	Velocity of impulses
            c.	Mentation changes
            d.	Thermoregulation changes
    D.	Special Considerations in Assessment
        1.	History
            a.	Can be unreliable historian
            b.	Underlying disease can change normal baseline for patient
                i.	mentation
                ii.	vital signs
    E.	Special Considerations in Management
        1.	Airway, Breathing, And Circulation Review
            a.	Mask seal with toothless patient
            b.	Cervical kyphosis
            c.	Oxygen saturation can quickly deteriorate
        2.	Circulation
            a.	Patients with chronic hypertension may have higher blood pressure value needs to achieve the same level of end organ perfusion than other patients
            b.	Patient may be in shock with blood pressure above 100 mmHg
            c.	Modest amounts of blood loss can lead to shock
                i.	reduced blood volume
                ii.	possible anemia
            d.	Patient is less able to tolerate excessive fluids
                i.	possible anemia
                ii.	possible electrolyte alterations

IV.   Cognitively Impaired Patient Trauma
    A.   Incidence
        1.   Mortality/morbidity
            a.   Accidental
            b.   Intentional
        2.   Risk factors
        3.   Prevention
    B.   Types of Cognitive Impairment
    C.   Challenges With Cognitive Impaired Patients
        1.   Ability of individual to communicate complaints
        2.   Unreliable historian
        3.   Unusual presentation of common disorders
        4.   Reduced pain threshold
        5.   Consent to treat complications
    D.   Special Considerations in Assessment
        1.   Level of development
            a.   5th or 6th grade level is common
            b.   Use open-ended questions to assess development
            c.   Particular difficulty with time and causality concepts
        2.   Communication ability assessment
            a.   How does patient normally communicate?
            b.   How aware are they of environment?
            c.   What are usual motor skills and level of activity?
            d.   Use a high-function concept and have them repeat it back
        3.   Assess/determine hearing and sight problems
        4.   Take vital signs when patient is calm
        5.   Typically helpful to have a caregiver present during physical exam.

Trauma
Environmental Emergencies

AEMT Education Standard

Applies fundamental knowledge to provide basic and selected advanced emergency care and transportation based on assessment findings for an acutely injured patient.

AEMT-Level Instructional Guideline

The AEMT Instructional Guidelines in this section include all the topics and material at the EMT level.

Trauma
Multiple-System Trauma

AEMT Education Standard

Applies fundamental knowledge to provide basic and selected advanced emergency care and transportation based on assessment findings for an acutely injured patient.

AEMT-Level Instructional Guideline

The AEMT Instructional Guidelines in this section include all the topics and material at the EMT level PLUS the following material:

I.   Kinematics of Trauma
    A.   Definition
        1.   Looking a trauma scene and attempting to determine what injuries might have resulted
        2.   Kinetic energy – function of weight of an item and its speed.
        3.   Blunt trauma
            a.   Objects collide during crashes
                i.   car with object
                ii.   victim with part of car
                iii.   organs collide inside body
            b.   Unbelted drivers and front seat passengers suffer multi-system trauma due to multiple collisions of the body and organs
            c.   Direction of the force has impact on type of injury
                i.   frontal impacts
                ii.   rear impacts
                iii.   side impacts
                iv.   rotational impacts
                v.   roll-overs
        4.   Deceleration injuries
        5.   Penetrating trauma
            a.   Types of bullets have affect
                i.   distance from shooter
                ii.   size of bullet
                iii.   fragmentation
                iv.   cavitation
            b.   Energy levels have effect
                i.   low energy -- stabbings
                ii.   medium energy -- handguns, some rifles
                iii.   high energy -- military weapons

      c.   Organs stuck have effect
             i.   head
             ii.   chest
             iii.   abdomen
             iv.   extremities

II.   Multi-System Trauma
    A.   Definition
        1.   Almost all trauma effects more than one system
        2.   Typically a patient considered to have "multi-trauma" has more than one major system or organ involved
            a.   Head and spinal trauma
            b.   Chest and abdominal trauma
            c.   Chest and multiple extremity trauma
        3.   Multi-trauma treatment will involve a team of physicians to treat the patient such as neurosurgeons, thoracic surgeons, and orthopedic surgeons
        4.   Multi-trauma has a high level of morbidity and mortality
    B.   The Golden Principles of Out-of-Hospital Trauma Care
        1.   Safety of patient and rescue personnel
        2.   Determination of additional resources
        3.   Kinematics
            a.   Mechanism of injury
            b.   High index of suspicion
        4.   Identify and manage life threats
        5.   Airway management while maintaining cervical spinal immobilization
        6.   Support ventilation and oxygenation
        7.   Control external hemorrhage
        8.   Basic shock therapy
            a.   Maintain normal body temperature
            b.   Splint musculoskeletal injuries
        9.   Maintain spinal immobilization on long board
            a.   Standing patients
            b.   Sitting patients
            c.   Rapid transport considerations
            d.   Prone patients
            e.   Supine patients
        10.   Transportation considerations
            a.   Golden period
            b.   Closest appropriate facility
            c.   'Platinum 10 Minutes'
        11.   Obtain medical history
        12.   Secondary survey after maintenance of life threats
        13.   "Do No Further Harm"
    C.   Critical Thinking in Multi-System Trauma Care
        1.   Airway, ventilation and oxygenation are key elements to success
            a.   Airways must be opened and clear throughout care

b.   Adequate ventilation must occur

c.   Oxygenation in multi-system trauma is high concentrations of oxygen

2.   Oxygenation cannot occur when patients are bleeding profusely

     a.   Stop arterial bleeding rapidly

     b.   Consider use of tourniquets in emergent, hostile or multiple patient situations where bleeding is considerable

3.   Sequence of treating patients

     a.   Not all treatments are linear. At times care must be adjusted depending on the needs of the patient.

     b.   Example:

          i.   control arterial bleeding in an awake patient first

          ii.   much care can be done en route

4.   Rapid transport is essential

     a.   The definitive care for multi-system trauma is surgery which can not be done in the field

     b.   On scene time is critical and should not be delayed

     c.   Rapid extraction is an important consideration

     d.   Use of ALS intercept and air medical resources in a multi-trauma patient should be highly considered

     e.   Early notification of hospital resources is essential once rapidly leaving the scene

     f.   Transport to the appropriate facility is critical

5.   Backboards

6.   Documentation and peporting

     a.   AEMTs are the only ones at the scene of multi-trauma patients

          i.   AEMTs are the eyes and ears of the physicians

          ii.   AEMTs need to re-create the scene

          iii.   important kinematics and mechanisms of injury are important to trauma teams

          iv.   changes in vital signs or assessment findings while en route are critical to report and document

7.   Personal safety

     a.   Most important when arriving on scene, and throughout care, an injured AEMT can not provide care

     b.   Be sure to assess your environment

          i.   passing automobiles

          ii.   hazardous situation

          iii.   hostile environments

          iv.   unsecured crime scenes

          v.   suicide patients who may become homicidal

8.   Experience

     a.   Newly licensed AEMTs who have not seen many multi-system trauma patients need to stick with the basics of life saving techniques

b.   Do not develop "tunnel" vision by focusing on patients who complain of lots of pain and are screaming for your help while other quiet patients who may be hypoxic or bleeding internally can not call out for help because of decreases in level of consciousness

c.   Be suspicious at trauma scenes, sometimes an obvious injury is not the critical cause one the potential for harm.

d.   Trauma care is a leading cause of death of young people. It is essential you keep important care principles in mind when providing care.

III.   Specific Injuries Related to Multi System Trauma
    A.   Blast Injuries
        1.   Types of blast injuries (explosions)
            a.   Release
                i.   blast waves
                ii.   blast winds
                iii.   ground shock
                iv.   heat
        2.   Pathophysiology
            a.   Blast waves when the victim is close to the blast cause disruption of major blood vessels, rupture of major organs, and lethal cardiac disturbances
            b.   Blast winds and ground shock can collapse buildings, cause trauma
        3.   Signs/symptoms
            a.   Hollow organs are injured first
            b.   Multi-system injury sign and symptom patterns
                i.   lungs
                ii.   heart
                iii.   major blood vessels
        4.   Management considerations in blast injuries
            a.   Multi-system trauma care
            b.   Immediate transport to appropriate facility
            c.   Multi-casualty care

Special Patient Populations
Obstetrics

AEMT Education Standard

Applies a fundamental knowledge of growth, development, aging, and assessment findings to provide basic and selected advanced emergency care and transportation for a patient with special needs.

AEMT-Level Instructional Guideline

The AEMT Instructional Guidelines in this section include all the topics and material at the EMT level.

Special Patient Populations
Neonatal Care

AEMT Education Standard

Applies a fundamental knowledge of growth, development, aging, and assessment findings to provide basic and selected advanced emergency care and transportation for a patient with special needs.

AEMT-Level Instructional Guideline

The AEMT Instructional Guidelines in this section include all the topics and material at the EMT level.

Special Patient Populations
Pediatrics

AEMT Education Standard

Applies a fundamental knowledge of growth, development, aging, and assessment findings to provide basic and selected advanced emergency care and transportation for a patient with special needs.

AEMT-Level Instructional Guideline

The AEMT Instructional Guidelines in this section include all the topics and material at the EMT level.

Special Patient Populations
Geriatrics

AEMT Education Standard

Applies a fundamental knowledge of growth, development, aging, and assessment findings to provide basic and selected advanced emergency care and transportation for a patient with special needs.

AEMT-Level Instructional Guideline

The AEMT Instructional Guidelines in this section include all the topics and material at the EMT level PLUS the following material:

I. Fluid Resuscitation in the Elderly
    A. Patients With Chronic Hypertension May Have Higher Blood Pressure Value Needs to Achieve the Same Level of End Organ Perfusion Than Other Patients
        1. Patient may be in shock with blood pressure above 100
        2. Modest amounts of blood loss can lead to shock
            a. Reduced blood volume
            b. Possible anemia
        3. Patient less able to tolerate excessive fluids
            a. Possible anemia
            b. Possible electrolyte alterations
        4. Hemodilution

Special Patient Populations
Patients With Special Challenges

AEMT Education Standard

Applies a fundamental knowledge of growth, development, aging, and assessment findings to provide basic and selected advanced emergency care and transportation for a patient with special needs.

AEMT-Level Instructional Guideline

The AEMT Instructional Guidelines in this section include all the topics and material at the EMT level PLUS the following material:

I.   Abuse and Neglect
       A.   Child Abuse
              1.   Types of abuse
              2.   Epidemiology
              3.   Assessment
                     a.   History or scene findings to concern for abuse or neglect
                     b.   Caregiver's behavior
                     c.   Physical findings
              4.   Management
                     a.   Reporting
                     b.   Safely transporting
                     c.   Role of child/adult protective services
              5.   Legal aspects
              6.   Documentation
       B.   Elder Abuse
              1.   Types of abuse
              2.   Epidemiology
              3.   Assessment
              4.   Management
              5.   Legal aspects
              6.   Documentation

II.   Homelessness/Poverty
       A.   Advocate for Patient Rights and Appropriate Care
       B.   Identify Facilities That Will Treat Regardless of Payment
       C.   Prevention Strategies Will Likely Be Absent, Increasing the Probability of Disease
       D.   Familiarity With Assistance Resources Offered in Community

III. Bariatric Patients
    A.   Increased Risk for
        1.   Diabetes
        2.   Hypertension
        3.   Heart disease
        4.   stroke
    B.   Patient Handling Issues
        1.   to prevent back injuries
        2.   to position the patient to breathe

IV. Technology Assisted/Dependent
    A.   Ventilation Devices
    B.   Apnea Monitoring/Pulse Oximetry
    C.   Long Term Vascular Access Devices
    D.   Dialysis Shunts
    E.   Nutritional Support
    F.   Elimination Diversion

V. Hospice Care and Terminally Ill
    A.   What Is Hospice?
        1.   Comfort care versus curative care
        2.   Terminally ill as verified by physician
        3.   Typically cancer, heart failure, Alzheimer's disease, AIDS
    B.   EMS Intervention
    C.   DNR Orders

VI. Tracheostomy Care
    A.   Tracheostomy: Surgical Opening From the Anterior Neck Into the Trachea
    B.   Consists of
        1.   Stoma
        2.   Outer cannula
        3.   Inner cannula
    C.   Routine Care
        1.   Keep stoma clean and dry
        2.   Change outer cannula as needed
        3.   Suction as needed
    D.   Acute Care

VII. Sensory Deficits
    A.   Sight
        1.   Service dogs
        2.   Allow patient to take your arm
        3.   Other

B.   Hearing Impaired
     1.   Hearing aid issues

     2.   Communication
          a.   face patient (so he can lip read)
          b.   lighted area
          c.   communicate by writing
          d.   obtain sign language interpreter
C.   Paralysis
     1.   Hemiplegia
     2.   Palsy
     3.   Paraplegia
     4.   Quadriplegia

VIII.   Homecare
     A.   Common for Patients Over Age 65
     B.   Various Reasons for Calls

IX.   Patient With Developmental Disability
     A.   Treat Like Any Other Patient
     B.   Family or Friends May Supply Additional Information
     C.   Take Special Care to Provide Explanations

EMS Operations
Principles of Safely Operating a Ground Ambulance

AMT Education Standard

Knowledge of operational roles and responsibilities to ensure patient, public, and personnel safety.

AMT-Level Instructional Guideline

The intent of this section is to give an overview of emergency response to ensure EMS personnel, patient, and other's safety during EMS operations. This does not prepare the entry-level student to be an experienced and competent driver.

Information related to the clinical management of the patient during emergency response is found in the clinical sections of the National EMS Education Standards and Instructional Guidelines for each personnel level.

The AEMT Instructional Guidelines in this section include all the topics and material at the EMR and EMT levels.

EMS Operations
Incident Management

Knowledge of operational roles and responsibilities to ensure patient, public, and personnel safety.

Information related to the clinical management of the patient within components of the Incident Management System (IMS) is found in the clinical sections of the National EMS Education Standards and Instructional Guidelines for each personnel level.

I.   Establish and Work Within the Incident Management System
    A.   Entry-Level Students Need to Be Certified in
        1.   ICS-100: Introduction to ICS, or equivalent
        2.   FEMA IS-700: NIMS, An Introduction
    B.   This Can Be Done as a Co requisite or Prerequisite or as Part of the Entry-Level Course

EMS Operations
Multiple Casualty Incidents

AEMT Education Standard

Knowledge of operational roles and responsibilities to ensure patient, public, and personnel safety.

AEMT-Level Instructional Guideline

The intent of this section is to give an overview of operating during a multiple casualty incident when a multiple casualty incident plan is activated.

Information related to the clinical management of the patients during a multiple casualty incident is found in the clinical sections of the National EMS Education Standards and Instructional Guidelines for each personnel level.

The EMT Instructional Guidelines in this section include all the topics and material at the EMR and EMT levels.

EMS Operations
Air Medical

Knowledge of operational roles and responsibilities to ensure patient, public, and personnel safety.

The intent of this section is to give an overview of operating safely in and around a landing zone during air medical operations and transport.

Information related to the clinical management of the patients during air medical operations is found in the clinical sections of the National EMS Education Standards and Instructional Guidelines for each personnel level.

I. Safe Air Medical Operations
- A. Types
  1. Rotorcraft
  2. Fixed wing
- B. Advantages
  1. Specialized care – skills, supplies, equipment
  2. Rapid transport
  3. Access to remote areas
  4. Helicopter hospital helipads
- C. Disadvantages
  1. Weather/environmental
  2. Altitude limitations
  3. Airspeed limitations
  4. Aircraft cabin size
  5. Terrain
  6. Cost
- D. Patient Transfer
  1. Interacting with flight personnel
  2. Patient preparation
  3. Scene safety
     - a. Securing loose objects
     - b. Approaching the aircraft
     - c. Landing zone
- E. Landing Zone Selection and Preparation
- F. Approaching the Aircraft
- G. Communication Issues

II.   Criteria for Utilizing Air Medical Response
       A.   Indications for Patient Transport
             1.   Medical
             2.   Trauma
             3.   Search and rescue
       B.   Activation
             1.   Local and State guidelines exist for air medical activation
                   a.   State statutes
                   b.   Administrative rules
                   c.   City/county/district ordinance standards

EMS Operations
Vehicle Extrication

AEMT Education Standard

Knowledge of operational roles and responsibilities to ensure patient, public, and personnel safety.

AEMT-Level Instructional Guideline

The intent of this section is to give an overview of vehicle extrication to ensure EMS personnel and patient safety during extrication operations. This does not prepare the entry-level student to become a vehicle extrication expert or technician.

Information related to the clinical management of the patient being cared for during vehicle extrication is found in the clinical sections of the National EMS Education Standards and Instructional Guidelines for each personnel level.

I. Safe Vehicle Extrication
   A. Role of EMS in Vehicle Extrication
      1. Provide patient care
      2. Perform simple extrication
   B. Personal Safety
      1. First priority for all EMS personnel
      2. Appropriate personal protective equipment for conditions
      3. Scene size-up
   C. Patient Safety
      1. Keep them informed of your actions
      2. Protect from further harm
   D. Situational Safety
      1. Control traffic flow
         a. Proper positioning of emergency vehicles
            i. upwind/uphill
            ii. protect scene
         b. Use of lights and other warning devices
         c. Setting up protective barrier
         d. Designate a traffic control person
      2. 360-degree assessment
         a. Downed electrical lines
         b. Leaking fuels or fluids
         c. Smoke or fire
         d. Broken glass
         e. Trapped or ejected patients
         f. Mechanism of injury

3. Vehicle stabilization
   a. Put vehicle in "park" or in gear
   b. Set parking brake
   c. Turn off vehicle ignition
   d. Cribbing/Chocking
   e. Move seats back and roll down windows
   f. Disconnect battery or power source
   g. Identify and avoid hazardous vehicle safety components
      i. seat belt pretensioners
      ii. undeployed air bags
      iii. other
4. Unique hazards
   a. Alternative-fuel vehicles
   b. Undeployed vehicle safety devices
   c. HAZMAT
5. Evaluate the need for additional resources
   a. Extrication equipment
   b. Fire suppression
   c. Law enforcement
   d. HAZMAT
   e. Utility companies
   f. Air medical
   g. Others
6. Extrication considerations
   a. Disentanglement of vehicle from patient
   b. Multi-step process
   c. Rescuer-intensive
   d. Equipment-intensive
   e. Time-intensive
   f. Access to patient
      i. simple
         a) try to open doors
         b) ask patient to unlock doors
         c) ask patient to lower windows
      ii. complex
      iii. tools
         a) hand
         b) pneumatic
         c) hydraulic
         d) other

E. Determine Number of Patients (Implement Local Multiple Casualty Incident Protocols If Necessary)

II. Use of Simple Hand Tools
   A. Hammer
   B. Center Punch

  C. Pry Bar
  D. Hack Saw
  E. Come-Along

III. Special Considerations for Patient Care
  A. Removing Patient
    1. Maintain manual cervical spine stabilization
    2. Complete primary assessment
    3. Provide critical interventions
  B. Assist With Rapid Extrication
  C. Move Patient, Not Device
  D. Use Sufficient Personnel
  E. Use Path of Least Resistance

EMS Operations
Hazardous Materials Awareness

AEMT Education Standard

Knowledge of operational roles and responsibilities to ensure patient, public, and personnel safety.

AEMT-Level Instructional Guideline

Information related to the clinical management of the patient exposed to hazardous materials is found in the clinical sections of the National EMS Education Standards and Instructional Guidelines for each personnel level.

I.   Risks and Responsibilities of Operating in a Cold Zone at a Hazardous Material or Other Special Incident
      A.   Entry-Level Students Need to Be Certified in:
            1.   Hazardous Waste Operations and Emergency Response (HAZWOPER) standard, 29 CFR 1910.120 (q)(6)(i) -First Responder Awareness Level
      B.   This Can Be Done as a Co requisite or Prerequisite or as Part of the Entry-Level Course

EMS Operations
Mass Casualty Incidents Due to Terrorism and Disaster

AEMT Education Standard

Knowledge of operational roles and responsibilities to ensure patient, public, and personnel safety.

AEMT-Level Instructional Guideline

The intent of this section is to give an overview of operating during a terrorist event or during a natural or manmade disaster.

Information related to the clinical management of patients exposed to a terrorist event is found in the clinical sections of the National EMS Education Standards and Instructional Guidelines for each personnel level.

I. Risks and Responsibilities of Operating on the Scene of a Natural or Man-Made Disaster
    A. Role of EMS
        1. Personal safety
        2. Provide patient care
        3. Initiate/operate in an incident command system (ICS)
        4. Assist with operations
    B. Safety
        1. Personal
            a. First priority for all EMS personnel
            b. Appropriate personnel protective equipment for conditions
            c. Scene size-up
            d. Time, distance, and shielding for self-protection
            e. Emergency responders are targets
            f. Dangers of the secondary attack
        2. Patient
            a. Keep them informed of your actions
            b. Protect from further harm
            c. Signs and symptoms of biological, nuclear, incendiary, chemical and explosive (B-NICE) substances
            d. Concept of "greater good" as it relates to any delay
            e. Treating terrorists/criminals

3.   360-degree assessment and scene size-up
     a.   Outward signs and characteristics of terrorist incidents
     b.   Outward signs of a weapons of mass destruction (WMD) incident
     c.   Outward signs and protective actions of biological, nuclear, incendiary, chemical, and explosive (B-NICE) weapons
4.   Determine number of patients (implement local multiple-casualty incident (MCI) protocols as necessary)
5.   Evaluate need for additional resources
6.   EMS operations during terrorist, weapons of mass destruction, disaster events
     a.   All hazards safety approach
     b.   Initially distance from scene and approach when safe
     c.   Ongoing scene assessment for potential secondary events
     d.   Communicate with law enforcement at the scene of an armed attack
     e.   Initiate or expand incident command system as needed
     f.   Perimeter use to protect rescuers and public from injury
     g.   Escape plan and a mobilization point at a terrorist incident
7.   Care of emergency responders on scene
     a.   Safe use of an auto injector for self and peers
     b.   Safe disposal of auto injector devices after activation

www.ingramcontent.com/pod-product-compliance
Lightning Source LLC
Chambersburg PA
CBHW080658190526

45169CB00006B/2170